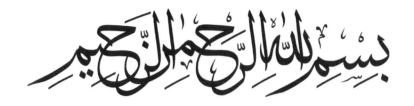

Islamic Cupping & Hijamah: A Complete Guide

By Dr Feroz Osman-Latib

Print Version

ISBN-10: 0-9911455-0-X
ISBN-13: 978-0-9911455-0-8

EDI Publishers
11 Mandrill Street
Lenasia 1827, South Africa
www.edipublishers.co.za
email: info@edipublishers.co.za

Ordering Information:
Quantity sales. Special discounts are available on quantity purchases by bookstore, associations, and others. For details, contact the publisher at the address above.

Contents

4

Foreword

This is one of the first books explaining cupping in such detail, it will benefit the patient and the practitioner to understand all the details of Hijamah.

Thus this book is a basic hand book on the practice of Hijamah for the layman and the medical practitioner.

Certain sections, only the one with good medical knowledge will benefit whilst the layman can draw information from other parts.

Many answers to commonly asked questions are well documented. Questions such as:-

1) Who should practice Hijamah?
2) The Shaari status of Hijamah?
3) Who should have Hijamah done?
4) When should Hijamah be done?
5) What to do after Hijamah?
6) and How it is basically done?

One can safely conclude that this is a highly skilled procedure to be done by an expert.

Also it is recommended, not jurisprudically Sunnat.

May Allaah reward Dr Feroz Latib for explaining this matter adequately and May Allaah continue using him for Deen.

A.H. Elias (Mufti)
May Allaah be with him
1434 - 2013

Preface

"Indeed the best of remedies you have is hijama"
- *Saheeh al-Bukhari (5371)*

All Praise is due to Allaah who gave us the Deen of Islaam and perfected it for us until the day of Qiyaamah. All praise is due to Allaah whom we cannot praise in the manner that He should be praised, He is as He has praised Himself. All praise is due to Allaah who sent our Noble Nabi Muhammad (SAW) as a mercy and guidance for all mankind.

Allaah Subhanahu wa Ta'aala has chosen mercy for His creation, and because of this, His commands and the life shown to us by His Ambiyaa (AS) encompass all that is beneficial for the spiritual, physical and social aspects of a human being, and society in general. Islaam itself places great emphasis on good health and physical fitness as this allows for the performance of Ibaadat and other acts that are meritorious in the eyes of Allaah. For this reason there are numerous Ahadeeth related to good health, the treatment of illness, the use of herbal substances etc. Entire books have been devoted to these topics, and amongst these writings perhaps the most famous are the Ahadeeth regarding honey, hijamah and habbatul barakah (black seed); as a result these three find common use amongst faithful Muslims the world over who adopt it for general health and the treatment of many, if not all medical conditions.

When one examines the Ahadeeth closely however, one realizes that there is a deeper layer that alludes to the treatment, whether it be hijamah, black seed, honey or any other treatment, being prescribed on the basis of "differentiation" which in turn requires sound medical knowledge. **From other Ahadeeth the Fuqahaa also deduce that one should visit a doctor who is an "expert" in their field.**

This brings to mind a wise saying that is quoted often in the books of our great scholars:

"Half a doctor is a danger to your life, and half a scholar is a danger to your faith"

The truth is that Hijamah is a medical procedure that should be performed by someone who has sound medical knowledge and is able to understand not only how to perform the procedure but when to do so, who to do it for, and when not to perform it.

The scholars of Islaam also advise that administering medicine requires medical expertise and should not be done by the layperson. Therefore, with regard to any medical treatment recommended by Rasulullaah (Sallallaahu Álayhi Wasallam), due to health and medical intricacies as well as most country laws that define the scope of practice of medicine and medical procedures, one must exercise caution and consult with a physician who is a qualified expert in that field. Similarly, **with regard to Hijamah, although it is strongly recommended by Rasulullaah (Sallallaahu Álayhi Wasallam) in numerous Ahaadeeth,** it will be necessary to consult with a qualified practitioner before undergoing cupping and then have it performed by one who has adequate medical training. This may be a medical practitioner or a practitioner of complementary and alternative medicine, who is duly qualified and registered with the relevant authority in that country to practice.

By doing so, one will gain the benefits of Hijamah without the inherent harm that exists in practicing Hijamah without complete knowledge of its intricacies. **This is one of the fundamental reasons why I have written this book, for the patient and practitioner alike to understand all the details regarding hijamah, so that it can be a means of cure and not a means of sickness.** Many will not understand this, as they believe that "cupping" or Hijamah must be beneficial at all times, since it is "Sunnah". This view is not correct and is not supported by the Ahadeeth either. **Hijamah when done at its appropriate time and for the right person who is in the condition suited to Hijamah will enable healing and cure for that person.**

I have been studying and teaching various aspects of complementary medicine for the past 18 years, including acupuncture, Chinese herbal medicine, chiropractic, laser therapy etc. I have a formal qualification from the Australian College of Natural Medicine where I specialized in Chinese Medicine and Acupuncture. I completed my internship at the Guangxi University Hospital in Nanning, China where I also received additional training in gynecology and pediatrics. I have taught at the South Australian College of Natural Medicine and also at the

University of the Western Cape in South Africa. Together with teaching, delivering seminars and having served at the Allied Health Professions Council of South Africa I have been practicing and teaching hijamah/cupping for the last 15 years.

In this time I have heard of many irresponsible practices being performed in the name of Hijamah, these have often led to many side-effects including but not limited to miscarriages, severe blood loss, permanent scarring etc. that can be experienced when Hijamah is done incorrectly and inappropriately.

Many well-meaning individuals have also sprung up in numerous countries who aggressively advertise Hijamah and perform it whilst ignoring its most basic principles, some doing it solely for monetary incentive. They seek to profit both from people's desire to practice on the "Sunnah", and the hope that the sick hold for finding a cure for their ailments. As a result of being ignorant of the finer details of Hijamah, they end up doing more harm than good.

It is my hope that by writing this guide, patients and practitioners alike will have adequate knowledge to use hijamah properly and gain the true benefits in this form of treatment, which when done correctly is like no other in terms of its healing effects on the body. **Those contemplating having it done will have a better understanding of when, how and if it should be performed in their case,** and those performing it will do so with sound knowledge and eliminate the serious side-effects inherent in its incorrect practice. They will then serve as a means for bringing this "Sunnah" treatment to many who are desperately in need of it.

The book is a complete guide to the basis and practice of Hijamah for the layperson and interested medical professionals. It discusses all the aspects of Hijamah in detail, but since it is primarily meant for the public who want to be educated about Hijamah, it excludes how to perform the procedure and also does not provide details on treating specific illnesses with Hijamah. I have included this practitioner level information in my Hijamah Treatment Guide for Practitioners, which is a series of manuals that detail exactly how to use Hijamah in the treatment of hundreds of health conditions and disorders, it includes procedures, special Hijamah points, diagnostic and differentiation methods, as well as ancillary therapeutic methods and is available at this link:
www.hijamahbook.com/treatment

Dr Feroz Osman-Latib
www.DrLatib.com
Twitter: @DrLatib

Introduction

Hijamah (حِجَامَة) comes from the Arabic root word حَجَم which means "to diminish in volume", and refers to the reduction in blood volume or to the vacuum effect used to draw blood from the body. In the case of the Ahaadeeth (sayings of the Nabi [SAW]) regarding hijamah it refers to the drawing of blood from the body for therapeutic purposes, either to maintain health in the case of one who is not sick or to cure a specific illness or ailment.

The vacuum or sucking effect can be achieved by many different methods including sucking with the mouth directly over a cut or wound (as in the case of poisonous bites), using a leech to draw blood, the use of instruments such as animal horns as was done in ancient times, or the more modern methods of using bamboo, glass or plastic "cups", either with fire or a pump mechanism.

The practice of applying a partial vacuum by these means causes the tissues beneath the cup to be drawn up and swell, thereby increasing blood flow to the affected area. This enhanced blood flow draws impurities and toxins away from the nearby tissues and organs towards the surface for elimination via the break in the skin layer created through the incisions made prior to the application of the "cup" or similar device.

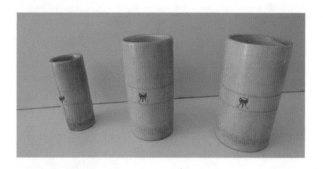

Bamboo cups were popular in Traditional Chinese Cupping before the arrival of plastic and glass cups. Many practitioners still prefer to use bamboo cups as they can be infused with an herbal decoction before application. Today it is not preferred for wet cupping as one cannot see the amount of blood being cupped and they are also impossible to sterilize.

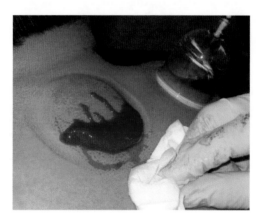

Nowadays plastic cups are commonly used for the cupping procedure and represent a safe and affordable method of creating the vacuum needed. These cups however must be disposed of after therapy, as the valve mechanism cannot be adequately sterilized.

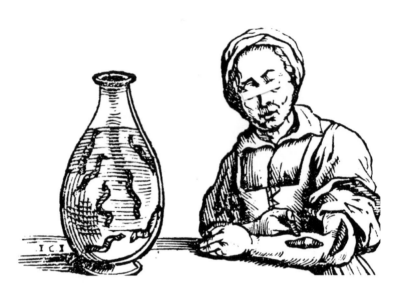

Leeches were also commonly used for drawing blood and have been approved by the FDA in the US for use in plastic and reconstructive surgery. These medicinal leeches are valued because while drawing blood they release natural anticoagulant and anesthetic substances and are therefore able to efficiently restore blood flow. Some cupping clinics employ the use of medicinal leeches and while it may be unpleasant it is in fact a safer and preferred option, which also leaves less scarring.

Cupping, Hijamah or Bloodletting

Though حجامة is commonly translated as "cupping" amongst English speakers, this is not an accurate translation because cupping in the modern sense can refer to both "dry" (where no blood is removed) and "wet" forms (which is حجامة). Cupping is the practice of using cups, which can be of different materials, to create suction at the skin level in order to draw blood to the surface, which may then be removed in the case of "wet" cupping.

Even amongst those who practice cupping, "wet" cupping is regarded the curative modality whereas dry cupping (in which no blood is removed), is a "relaxation therapy" and often practiced as part of relaxation massage techniques. Chinese medicine practitioners however do use dry cupping in order to "invigorate blood flow" in cases of blood "stasis", yet this is a relatively new phenomenon in Chinese medicine where practitioners especially in western countries avoid drawing of blood.

While dry cupping has its uses, it is limited in its therapeutic effectiveness since the blood is drawn to the surface but not released, hence the effect of improving blood flow as well as release of some heat through the pores is achieved, but it is a temporary effect.

"Bloodletting" is the preferred term for حجامة and will be used throughout this book as it is more true to the meaning of Hijamah as implied by the Hadeeth. This is more so relevant since "cups" or similar instruments are not always used in the Hijamah procedure, as even an incision in the right part of the body intended to release blood from that area can be considered Hijamah, so can the use of leeches to draw blood. Both do not involve the use of cups, but are true to the essence of Hijamah. In fact there are Ahadeeth where the "blade of the Hajjaam" is mentioned as having the cure and is a indication that the act of releasing blood is the curative factor in Hijamah and not which instrument is used to draw the blood.

In keeping with this understanding, the one who performs Hijamah will be referred to as the حَجَّام (Hajjaam) in this book.

History of Hijamah

It is recorded in the books of Ahadeeth that amongst other things, such as the use of the turban and miswak, hijamah was a practice of every Nabi (AS). Considering that the Quran clearly states that every nation was sent a guide, and the fact that at least 124 000 Ambiyaa (AS) were sent to this world, Hijamah as a treatment is to be found throughout the world as a result of this long history of continuous use. Indeed historical texts prove that this is the case with depictions of cupping equipment being seen on ancient stone tablets and markings from archeological findings throughout the world.

The earliest historical evidence of the use of Hijamah is from the ancient Egyptians. One of the oldest Egyptian medical textbooks, written in approximately 1550 BC, describes "bleeding" used to 'remove pathogens from the body'. It is evident that bloodletting was considered a remedy for almost every type of disease as well as an important means of preserving good health and life.

Hippocrates and Galen were also great advocates of Hijamah. In Hippocrates' time bloodletting was topological and not used in terms of the theory of the 4 humors. Specific points were bled for specific illnesses. Galen explains that the principle indication for bloodletting is to eliminate residues or divert blood from one part of the body to another. His approach was based on two key Unani concepts prevalent at the time. **First, that blood did not circulate well in the body, and that it eventually**

went stagnant until it was "let out". Secondly, the concept of the balance of the four humors (blood, phlegm, black bile and yellow bile) was the source of health or illness, in which case bloodletting is used to bring about balance between these humors. Mapping out the blood vessels of the body, Galen would cut his patients in different areas; depending on what area he wanted to treat.

In the middle east region we find that the practice of Hijamah was already present before the arrival of the final Rasul (SAW) and the final Nabi (SAW) both encouraged and used it himself on many occasions. **Ibn Sina, the famous Muslim physician said: 'Hijamah is not preferred in the beginning or the end of the month. It is preferred in the middle of the month when the substances (of the constitution or the condition) accumulate and become agitated.**

The Talmud included rules for days where bloodletting could be practiced and early Christian writings also outlined which days were the best for bloodletting therapy.

In the East, Bloodletting and wet cupping was always an integral part of the medical practices, and remains so to this day. The ancient Chinese medical text which is widely regarded as the oldest medical text in existence, the *Nei Jing*, or *Inner Classic* says that:

"if there is stagnation it must be first be resolved through bloodletting before the application of acupuncture or moxibustion."

Another ancient Chinese medical text the *Su Wen* gives detailed instructions for piercing combined with bloodletting but forbidding the letting of blood in certain seasons.

The Su Wen states:

"When heaven is warm and when the sun is bright,
then the blood in man is rich in liquid
and the protective qi (energy/lifeforce) is at the surface
Hence the blood can be drained easily, and the qi can be made to move on easily..."

Some researchers believe that acupuncture actually began as bloodletting, with sharp objects being used to bleed the acupuncture points before the widespread use of needles to perform acupuncture. This is also evidenced by depictions of ancient "needles" which were more akin to bleeding instruments than the fine acupuncture needles in use today.

The Lingshu (Spiritual Pivot) and its companion volume, the Suwen (Simple Questions), written around 100 B.C., established the fundamentals of traditional Chinese medical ideas and acupuncture therapy. Originally, there was a set of 9 acupuncture needles, which included the triangular lance, sword-like flat needles, and fairly large needles. Regarding the fourth needle, which has a tubular body and lance-like tip, the text states: "This can be used to drain fevers, to draw blood, and to exhaust chronic diseases." The seventh needle is described as being hair fine (corresponding to modern acupuncture needles); it is said to "control fever and chills and painful rheumatism in the luo channels." In modern practice, using the lance as a means to treat chronic diseases has been marginalized (except to treat acute flare-ups of chronic ailments), while the applications of the hair-fine needle has been greatly expanded beyond malarial fevers and muscle and joint pain.

Traditional Chinese Medicine and Acupuncture practitioners still use bleeding therapies though it is more commonly practiced in China than by western practitioners due to concerns about infection and the general dislike for dealing with blood in the acupuncture clinic.

North American natives are reported to have used buffalo horns for wet cupping. The horns were hollowed with a small hole at the top through which the cupper would suck the air out of, in order to create a vacuum in the horn which would then pull up the blood from the incisions previously made with a blade.

Buffalo horns are also reported as being used for Hijamah during the Babylon - Assyrian Empire (stretching from Iraq to the Mediterranean).

Bloodletting became widespread during the middle ages and surprisingly, became a practice common to barbers who would display a "bloodletting pole" outside their establishment to indicate that they practiced bloodletting.

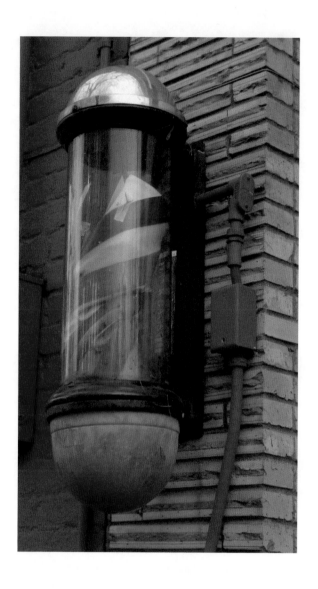

In this way it also became widespread in the US due to colonial influence from Europe and as a matter of fact, George Washington, the first U.S. president, died after having close to 4 liters of blood removed from his body on the same day as a treatment for an infection!

The traditional principles of Hijamah were largely being ignored during this time with the procedure being carried out incorrectly by barbers who had no medical knowledge and was therefore resulting in a large number of adverse effects and even many unnecessary deaths.

In Europe, the main process of bloodletting in the 19th century as performed by those in the medical establishment included the use of leeches to drain blood from a patient. France reportedly imported approximately 40 million leeches for the purpose of bloodletting during this period.

In Finland, medicinal bleeding has been practiced at least since the 15th century, and it is still done traditionally in saunas. Cups made of cow's horns were commonly used. These had a valve mechanism in it to create the negative pressure within the cup for suction to take place. (Wet cupping is still commonly used in Finland as a complementary/alternative medicine.)

By the mid to late 1800's however, bloodletting was sharply criticized by the medical fraternity and had fallen away as a popular method. Because of the procedure not being practiced correctly it was becoming responsible for a large number of deaths and therefore was increasingly being discredited by modern medicine, the newly established scientific model of medicine also began discrediting all other previously established traditional therapies in order to gain medical dominance.

There were valid concerns regarding the practice as well and in 1828, Pierre Charles Alexandre Louis openly criticized bloodletting for the treatment of diseases. His research found that in patients with pneumonia, 44% of those who were bled within the first four days died, compared with 25% of those patients who were bled later in their illness. He deduced that bloodletting was not useful in the treatment of pneumonia.

Bloodletting managed to survive however into the first part of the 20th century; it was even recommended in a 1923 edition of a textbook called *The Principles and Practice of Medicine*. During those days, there were four main bloodletting methods practiced by physicians. The first was the continued use of leeches as a bloodletting modality. The second was bleeding of superficial arteries. The third was phlebotomy (also known as "breathing a vein") where a large external vein would be cut in order to draw blood and the last was scarification – a method which involved using tools to make multiple incisions in the skin from which blood was drawn through "cupping".

As the 20th century brought new medical knowledge, technology and scientific research based validation (and negation) of medical practices, bloodletting died out in modern medicine in the western world almost entirely within a few decades. It remained very much still a part of Chinese (and Japanese) Medical therapy, though practitioners trained outside of China or Japan were reluctant to perform the procedure. It also remained in use in the Muslim world including the Middle East and countries with larger Muslim populations such as Indonesia, Malaysia etc.

In the past 20 to 30 years it has found a tremendous resurgence amongst Muslim communities living in other parts of the world as well, with courses being offered to both medical practitioners and the public in some countries like the UK.

In most western countries however like the US, Canada and Australia, medical law does not permit the practice of Hijamah by a non-medical trained individual though the practice may still exist informally amongst certain Muslim communities.

Since it involves piercing of the skin and exposure to blood and other body fluids and there is therefore a high risk of spreading of infections such as HIV and Hepatitis, not to mention the possibility of serious side effects, authorities in these countries have appropriately seen fit to legislate its use to qualified and registered health practitioners such as acupuncturists, medical practitioners etc.

Ahadeeth on Hijamah

The books of Ahaadeeth, which are the sayings and also the practices of the Nabi Muhammad (SAW) as recorded by his illustrious companions (RA) are replete with the mention of Hijamah describing its virtues and giving advice about when it is to be performed etc. In this section I will mention only the Ahadeeth regarding its virtues and also the hadith indicating the permissibility of paying a fee for the treatment. The Ahadeeth regarding payment are mentioned because there are many of the belief that there should be no payment for Hijamah whereas this is against the Sunnah of the Nabi (SAW). Other Ahadeeth regarding the specific matters of Hijamah will be discussed in their relevant chapters.

Virtues of Hijamah

*Jabir bin Abdullaah (RA) relates that he heard Rasulullaah (SAW) saying: "If there is any good in your treatments **it is in the blade of the Hajjaam**, a drink of honey or branding by fire (cauterization), whichever suits the ailment, and I do not like to be cauterized" (Bukhari and Muslim)*

Asim b. 'Umar b. Qatada reported: There came to our house 'Abdullaah and another person from amongst the members of the household who complained of a wound. Jabir said: What ails you? He said: There is a wound which is very painful for me, whereupon he said: Lad, bring to me a cupper. He said: 'Abdullaah, what do you intend to do with the Hajjaam? I said: I would get this wound cupped.

He said: By Allaah, even the touch of a fly or cloth causes me pain (and cupping) would thus cause me (unbearable) pain. And when he saw him feeling pain (at the idea of Hijamah), he said: I heard Allaah's Rasul (may peace be upon him) as saying: **If there is any effective remedy amongst your remedies, these are (three): Hijamah, drinking of honey and cauterization with the help of fire.** *Allaah's Rasul (may peace be upon him) had said: As for myself I do not like cauterization. The Hajjaam was called and he cupped him and he was all right. (Sahih Muslim 26:5468)*

Narrated By Abu Hurayrah (RA): Abu Hind cupped the Nabi (SAW) in the middle of his head. The Nabi (SAW) said: Banu Bayadah, marry Abu Hind (to your daughter), and ask him to marry (his daughter) to you. He said: **The best thing by which you treat yourself is Hijamah.** *(Abu Dawud 5:2097)*

Narrated By Abu Hurayrah: The Nabi (pbuh) said: **The best medical treatment you apply is Hijamah.** *(Abu Dawud 22:3848)*

Abu Hurairah (RA) narrates that Rasulullaah (SAW) said: "**Whoever has hijamah done on the 17th, 19th or 21st of the month, it will be for him a cure from every illness**" (Sahih Al-Jaami' 5968)

Abu Hurairah (RA) narrates that Rasulullaah (SAW) said: "Jibra'eel conveyed to me that **the best amongst the things that mankind uses for treatment is hijamah**" (Sahih Al-Jaami 213)

Abdullaah ibn Abbas (RA) reported that the Rasul (SAW) said, "I did not pass by an angel from the angels on the night journey except that they all said to me: **Upon you is Hijamah, O Muhammad.**" [Saheeh Sunan ibn Maajah (3477).

In the narration reported by Abdullaah ibn Mas'ud (RA) the angels said, "**Oh Muhammad, order your Ummah (nation) with Hijamah.**" [Saheeh Sunan Tirmidhi (3479)]

Rasulullaah (Sallallaahu Álayhi Wasallam) said, 'Jibraaeel (Álayhis salaam) **repeatedly emphasized upon me to resort to Hijamah** to the extent that I feared that Hijamah will be made compulsory.' (Jamúl Wasaail p. 179).

Rasulullaah (Sallallaahu Álayhi Wasallam) praised a person who performs Hijamah, saying **it removes blood, lightens the back and sharpens the eyesight** (Jamúl Wasaail p. 179)

Hadhrat Abu Kabsha (Radhiallaahu Ánhu) narrates that Rasulullaah (Sallallaahu Álayhi Wasallam) used to undergo cupping on the head and between his shoulders and he used to say, '**Whosoever removes this blood, it will not harm him that he does not take any other medical treatment.**' (Mishkãt p. 389)

Reasons for having Hijamah

Besides the general effects of Hijamah in improving and maintaining good health, especially in the hot regions, the Nabi (SAW) also used and recommended Hijamah for specific illnesses.

Injury

Jaabir ibn Abdullaah (RA) reported that the Rasul (SAW) fell from his horse onto the trunk of a palm tree and dislocated his foot. Waki' (RA) said, "Meaning the Rasul (SAW) **was cupped on (his foot) for bruising.**" [Saheeh Sunan ibn Maajah (2807)].

Headaches

Salma (RA), the servant of the Rasul (SAW) said, **"Whenever someone would complain of a headache to the Rasul of Allaah (SAW), he (SAW) would advise them to perform Hijamah.**" [Saheeh Sunan abi Dawud (3858)].

Sihr (black magic)

Ibn al-Qaiyum (RA) mentions that the Rasul (SAW) **was cupped on his head when he was afflicted with sihr** and that it is from the best of cures for this if performed correctly. [Zaad al Ma'aad (4/125-126)].

Poison

Abdullaah ibn Abbas (RA) reported that a Jewish woman gave poisoned meat to the Rasul (SAW) so he (SAW) sent her a message saying, "What caused you to do that?" She replied, "If you really are a Nabi then Allaah will inform you of it and if you are not then I would save the people from you!" **When the Rasul (SAW) felt pain from it, he (SAW) performed Hijamah. Once he travelled while in Ihram and felt that pain and hence performed hijamah.** [Ahmed (1/305) the Hadeeth is Hasan].

These four conditions mentioned in the Ahadeeth for which the Nabi (SAW) had Hijamah done give us an indication as to what type of diseases Hijamah is useful for viz.:

1.External injuries
2.Internal disorders which are either due to heat, poor circulation or build up of toxins
3.Sihr (black magic)
4.Poison (this can also be natural poisons such as heavy metal toxicity etc.)

(A detailed list of more than 150 conditions that can be treated with Hijamah, together with the method of treating of them are discussed in greater detail in my Hijamah Treatment Guide for Practitioners, if you are a practitioner of Hijamah or intend becoming one, I suggest getting the guide which is available at this link: www.hijamahbook.com/treatment)

Paying the Hajjaam

Ibn 'Umar RadiyAllaahu 'Anhu reports: "Rasulullaah SallAllaahu 'Alayhi Wasallam called a hajjaam, who treated Rasulullaah SallAllaahu 'Alayhi Wasallam. Rasulullaah SallAllaahu 'Alayhi Wasallam inquired from him what tax or duty did he have to pay daily? He replied, three saa'. Rasulullaah SallAllaahu 'Alayhi Wasallam had it reduced to two saa', **and gave him his remuneration**". (Tirmidhi 49:004)

Anas RadiyAllaahu'Anhu was asked regarding the payment to a hajjaam. (Is it permissible or not?) Anas RadiyAllaahu 'Anhu replied: "Rasulullaah SallAllaahu 'Alayhi Wasallam took the treatment of Hijamah which was administered by Abu Taybah RadiyAllaahu 'Anhu, **he was given two saa' food** (in a narration it is mentioned that dates were given), and Sayyidina Rasulullaah SallAllaahu'Alayhi Wasallam interceded on his behalf to his master that the stipulated amount he was responsible for be made less. He also said this, that Hijamah is the best of medicine".(Tirmidhi 49:001)

'Ali RadiyAllaahu 'Anhu reports: "Rasulullaah SallAllaahu 'Alayhi Wasallam once took the treatment of Hijamah **and asked me to pay its fees. I paid the hajjaam his fees**". (Tirmidhi 49:002)

Ibn 'Abbaas RadiyAllaahu 'Anhu said that Rasulullaah SallAllaahu 'Alayhi Wasallam took the treatment of Hijamah on both sides of his neck and between his shoulders, and **paid the hajjaam his fees. If it had been haraam, he would not have paid it. (**Tirmidhi 49:003)

The issue of Ijazah

Some books vehemently oppose the performing of Hijamah without "Ijazah", which literally means "permission" and refers to the granting of such permission by a teacher or sheikh to a student that he deems fit to perform the practice. This is a nonsensical idea and a clear error. If this were true then who gave "Ijazah" to the slave who performed Hijamah for the Nabi (SAW)? The fact is that Hijamah was already being practiced before Islaam, and in fact there is a reference to this in the hadith where the Nabi (SAW) says "the best of **your** medicine is Hijamah". Scholars mention that "your" in the hadith is an indication that this was already a practice of the people of Hijaz.

The truth is that "Ijazah" is not needed to perform Hijamah, but rather sound knowledge of its method and principles are needed. The benefits of Hijamah will be attained irrespective of whether the person performing it is a sheikh or even a Muslim. Yes, it is better that a pious Muslim practitioner performs the procedure but it is not an essential aspect of Hijamah or gaining is benefits.

Types of Hijamah / Bloodletting

There are a number of different methods and types of bloodletting and while the Hajjaam should know in detail which method is best, based on the patients health, the presenting ailment and general constitution, as well as geographic, seasonal and climatic factors, the patient should also be aware of these differences.

Hijamah in the condition of strength

The simplest method of Hijamah is that used for general health promotion and the Nabi (SAW) used the most common method. In this type of Hijamah there is no serious complaint by the patient that would warrant a special type of Hijamah or the use of "special" Hijamah points other than the standard points on the back, neck or head. This is traditionally termed as Hijamah-bi-Sihhat (Hijamah in the condition of health), many also refer to it as "sunnah cupping". Both terms are not correct however as the Rasul of Allaah (SAW) had cupping done both in health and as a treatment for particular pains and ailments, and it is also rare to find someone nowadays with absolutely no illness. I prefer the term Hijamah in strength, referring to performing Hijamah for someone who is of general good health and strength.

Such a patient may however complain of general symptoms such as a feeling of sluggishness, tiredness etc, they may also have a regular habit of

34

doing Hijamah and are aware of the benefits it has for them personally, or they are trying this method of health preservation for the first time under recommendation from their friends or acquaintances. Their general health is good, and very importantly their pulse is strong indicating a healthy amount of blood and also a good amount of heat in the blood. They may also be suffering from a constitutional blood or heat excess as is common in hot climates.

If the pulse is weak or deep then this type of Hijamah is not indicated as it means that there is deficient blood or the heat of the body is internal and not in the exterior parts of the body. (The method of feeling and interpreting the pulse is detailed in the Hijamah Treatment Guide for Practitioners)

In this type of Hijamah care is taken to observe the rules of Hijamah with regard to the condition of the patient, as well as the season, climate, day of the lunar month and time of the day in which Hijamah is performed as this greatly influences the nature of blood that will be removed. **Not observing these and performing this type of general Hijamah outside of its recommended times will not result in any benefit for the patient and will very often result in long term harm for the patients health.** This may not be apparent immediately after the procedure, but will be noticed in the months and even years to come afterward.

When applying Hijamah in the condition of strength the areas being cupped are standard, these are mentioned in the Ahadeeth:

35

Hadhrat Abu Kabsha (Radhiallaahu Ánhu) narrates that Rasulullaah (Sallallaahu Álayhi Wasallam) used to undergo cupping on the **head and between his shoulders** and he used to say, 'Whosoever removes this blood, it will not harm him that he does not take any other medical treatment.' (Mishkāt p. 389)

From examining the various Ahadeeth and by consensus of those experienced practitioners of Hijamah the areas used in this general form of Hijamah are;

For a man:

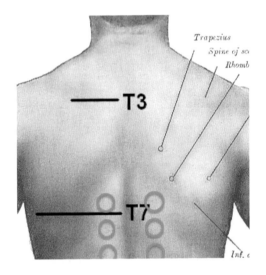

1. The area between the shoulder blades, most commonly in line with the inferior end of the scapula which is in line with the 7th thoracic vertebra. Sometimes other points lateral to the spinal column between the spinouts processes of the 6th to 9th thoracic vertebrae are used. This particular area is the best for performing general

Hijamah as it is the area where toxins and impurities in the blood accumulate and stagnate especially around the 17th. 19th and 21st of the month. In Traditional Chinese Medicine this point is regarded as the meeting point of the blood and is used for all blood disorders whether due to deficiency or excess.

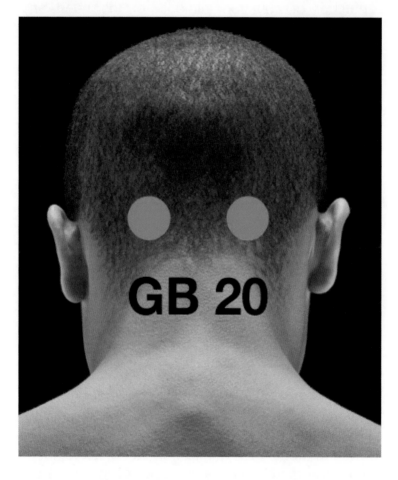

2. The occipital area of the neck in the recesses formed between the upper portion of the

sternocleidomastoid and the trapezius muscles. This is in the region of a commonly used acupuncture point called Feng Chi, which means "wind pool". It is believed that many pathogens enter the body at this area and that is why it is recommended to cover this area when it is cold or windy. Treating this area is helpful in resolving a number of common ailments of the head and neck, including headache, vertigo, pain/stiffness of neck, blurry vision, red/painful eyes, tinnitus, nasal obstruction, common cold, and rhinorrhea (runny nose, nasal discharge associated with allergies or hay fever or common cold). It's also very useful for insomnia, and tends to have a relaxing and balancing effect upon the nervous system.

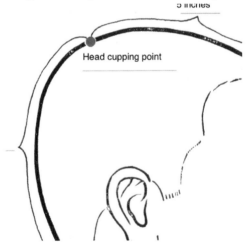

3. On the head in the midline, the exact point is normally directly above the apex of the ear as in the diagram below:

In Traditional medicine this point corresponds with the acupuncture point called Bai Hui, meaning a hundred convergences and is the meeting point of all the yang energy of the body. It is commonly used to treat all mental, emotional disorders, but also useful for headaches, epilepsy, neurological and endocrine disorders.

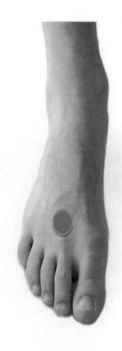

4. On the anterior aspect of the foot in a depression distal to the junction of the 2nd and 3rd metatarsal bones. This area is traditionally used to treat swelling, headache, dizziness / vertigo, abdominal

pain, bloating, constipation. It can also aid groundedness and focus and treat ADD/ADHD, mania, restlessness, palpitations and epilepsy.

In women the same areas are used except for the Hijamah point on the head but the quantity of blood removed is less. Note that women are not in need of regular Hijamah as they do release blood through the menses, if they have experienced menopause then it is fine to do as long as they are still strong and not suffering from blood deficiency in which case one must observe the rules of performing Hijamah in illness.

Days for performing Hijamah in strength

Anas ibn Maalik (RA) reported that the Rasul (SAW) said, **"Whoever wants to perform Hijamah then let him search for the 17th, 19th and 21st..."** [Saheeh Sunan ibn Maajah (3486)].

These are the generally accepted dates for Hijamah, irrespective of what day of the week they fall on, though there are other Ahadeeth that seem to prohibit having it done on particular days of the week, these Hadeeth are categorized as Daeef however and as such the days mentioned in them are not strictly prohibited, they are mentioned here for completeness:

Ibn Umar (RA) reported that the Rasul (SAW) said, "Hijamah on an empty stomach is best. In it is a cure and a blessing. It improves the intellect and the memory. So cup yourselves with the blessing of

Allaah on Thursday. Keep away from Hijamah on Wednesday, Friday, Saturday and Sunday to be safe. Perform Hijama on Monday and Tuesday for it is the day that Allaah saved Ayoub from a trial. He was inflicted with the trial on Wednesday. You will not find leprosy except (by being cupped) on Wednesday or Wednesday night." [Sunan ibn Maajah (3487)].

Ibn Umar (RA) reported that the Rasul (SAW) said, "Hijamah on an empty stomach is best. It increases the intellect and improves the memory. It improves the memory of the one memorising. So whoever is going to be cupped then (let it be) on a Thursday in the name of Allaah. Keep away from being cupped on a Friday, Saturday and Sunday. Be cupped on a Monday or Tuesday. Do not be cupped on a Wednesday because it is the day that Ayoub was befallen with a trial. You will not find leprosy except (by being cupped) on Wednesday or Wednesday night." [Sunan ibn Maajah (3488)].

In reconciling these it can be said that for Hijamah in strength, the dates are specified, they are the 17th, 19th or 21st of the lunar month and the best is when these dates coincide with a Monday, Tuesday or Thursday, though there is no prohibition for having this type of Hijamah done on any other day as long as it corresponds with the 17th, 19th and 21st.

(There is difference of opinion regarding the prohibition on particular days of the week, since another way of reconciling is considering that the Nabi of Allaah (SAW) in the above two Ahadeeth was

referring to that particular month in which the Hadeeth was narrated and referring directly to the days of that week and the week after. If Thursday was the 19th, then the previous Friday, Saturday and Sunday would be the 13th, 14th and 15th, and on these days of the Islaamic month it is mentioned that cupping should not be done, Monday and Tuesday would be the 16th and 17th which would be okay for cupping, since they are after the full moon. Wednesday being prohibited in this case would be the exact day of the year that corresponded with the illness of Nabi Ayyoob (AS), and Thursday being the ideal day to perform Hijamah.)

It is important to note that this type of Hijamah (i,.e Hijamah in strength / Sunnah Hijamah) should be performed only in the seasons of spring and summer. When the climate is hot. However, in places like Hejaz where it is hot throughout the year it can also be performed in the other seasons.

Further detail is discussed in the chapters on the guidelines for performing Hijamah.

Hijamah in illness

When a patient is complaining of a particular condition, i.e. they are not in good health, but suffering from a particular illness for which Hijamah is indicated then this is termed Hijama-bil-Mardh (Hijamah in illness).

In illness the rules of Hijamah are different. For this reason Imam Ahmad ibn Hanbal would have Hijamah at any time of the month and hour of the day as a result of the need of performing Hijamah due to illness. When performing Hijamah for a specific illness it should be done at those points of the body indicated for the illness and the rules of the amount of blood being removed etc. should be adhered to for maximum benefit. These are discussed in the Hijamah treatment guide. This type of Hijamah is very specialized and involves two major aspects, the correct selection of points (or superficial veins) to bleed and removing the correct amount of blood in order to effect cure of the patient's illness. It is also highly recommended to use herbal preparations in association with the Hijamah to address deficiencies/excesses present and treat cold or heat that is present.

Phlebotomy vs Hijamah

Phlebotomy is often confused with Hijamah yet the two are very different in their method and effect on the body. Phlebotomy is the bleeding of veins via the use of a hypodermic needle and results in releasing of blood from the inner parts of the body as opposed to the outer part which is achieved through traditional Hijamah. It will also be regarded as part of bloodletting, but not Hijamah, as there are significant differences in the use of these two types of bloodletting.

To understand the difference it is important to remember that the land of Hijaaz (where the Ahadeeth of Hijamah are reported) is hot. Hot and cold temperatures have different effects on the blood flow and distribution in the body. In hot countries, and other countries in the hot season, the blood and heat of the body flows more within the outer part of the body, and the inner parts remain cool and relatively deficient of blood. For this reason perspiration increases in summer, and because of the inner organs etc. being cooler, foods take longer to digest, and many summer-heat type illnesses occur. In cold countries, and in winter, the blood and heat of a person's body goes to the inner portions. As a result the digestive system is strengthened, more sleep is experienced, and food is digested easily.

For this reason rich foods digest easily in winter, and take more time in summer. This is also the reason honey; dates and other heat creating foods do not affect the people of Hijaaz. In Hijamah, the blood in the outer parts of the body is removed, and in Hijaaz the heat is more on the outer parts of the body, therefore, Hijamah is more beneficial in hot countries and hot climates. In phlebotomy blood is let from the hypodermic veins and reduces heat from the inner parts of the body, therefore it will not be beneficial in hot countries and climates and was hence not a practice of the Nabi (SAW).

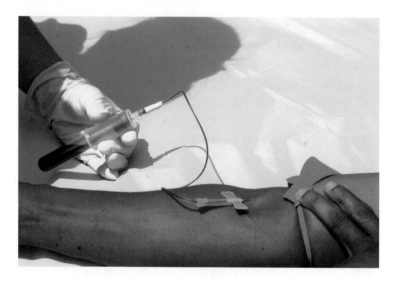

Drawing blood from the veins beneath the superficial skin layer is considered phlebotomy and does not have the same effect as traditional Hijamah

The effects of Hijamah on the body

The simplest explanation of Hijamah's effects is common in all cultures that perform Hijamah, viz. the removal of "bad" blood or impurities from the blood. This is a common theme whether it is from the Indians of North America to lay practitioners in western countries. Some may also use it for its ability to remove the effects of "sihr" or "black magic" as well as "nazr" or the "evil eye". The latter concepts are beyond the scope of this book but suffice to say that these are valid effects of Hijamah.

Common effects of Hijamah

1. Removal of "bad" blood or impurities from the blood
2. Treatment of Sihr or Nazr

There are other effects that are explained in more detail in a number of traditional medical systems as well as through modern scientific research. Understanding these is important as it allows for the correct selection and application of Hijamah techniques depending on the patient and the illness they are presenting with.

Amongst the traditional medical paradigms, Unani-Tibb and Traditional Chinese Medicine are the most detailed in terms of understanding why and how Hijamah works in maintaining health and treating illness. Unani-Tibb is practiced in the Graeco-Arab region as well as by Unani practitioners throughout the world. Traditional Chinese Medicine is practiced in the Asian regions and also by practitioners throughout the world and these two have similar philosophies with regards to the effect of Hijamah.

Unani-tibb is a form of traditional medicine widely practiced by Muslims and is largely based on the teachings of the Greek physician Hippocrates, and Roman physician Galen, which was developed into an elaborate medical System by Arab and Persian physicians, such as al-Razi, Ibn Sena, Al-Zahrawi, and Ibn Nafis. **Muslim practitioners are referred to as a Hakim, literally meaning "wise".**

Unani philosophy is based on the concept of the four humors: Phlegm (Balgham), Blood (Dam), Yellow bile (Ṣafrā') and Black bile (Saudā'). It maintains that disease occurs through imbalance, or contamination, of the 4 humors, or alternatively as a result of the body being weak. It is very much concerned with the temperament of the body and considers aspects such as heat, coolness, dryness, phlegm and moisture and how these cause and contribute to illness. **Bloodletting acts to remove contamination in the blood, rebalance the humors and draws excessive heat out of the body.** In the case of traditional Hijamah (as opposed to phlebotomy) this heat will be drawn from the <u>outer</u> parts of the body, though there are indirect effects on the internal organs and systems.

Contemporary Unani practitioners believe that Hijamah acts to draw inflammation and pressure away from the deep organs (especially the heart, brain, lungs, liver and kidneys) towards the skin. This facilitates the healing process. They also explain that this process strengthens the immune system, encouraging the optimum functioning of the body by assisting the actions of Physis. It diverts toxins and other harmful impurities from these vital organs towards the "less-vital skin", before expulsion. The blood that is diverted also then allows for a fresh 'stream' of blood to that area.

Effects of Hijamah as per Unani-Tibb

3. Diverts and expels toxins and harmful impurities from the vital organs
4. Removes excess blood
5. Removes excess heat from the blood and surface of the body
6. Draws inflammation away from the deeper organs
7. Assists the body's own healing abilities

Traditional Chinese Medicine(TCM) is similar to Unani-Tibb in its concept of "Humors", though in the case of TCM it is the balance of 5 phases/elements viz. water, fire, wood, earth and metal and their correspondences in the body. TCM however also adds the concept of proper movement and flow of blood and "qi" throughout the body. **Qi is the vital energy of the body that is responsible for directing all the body's functions.** It moves within the blood and it also moves the blood itself. Qi is present in different forms, it includes but is not limited to the energy of the heart and lungs as they contract and expand, the force of the muscles in the body that open and close the various sphincters and also allow for bodily movement. It is also responsible for many phenomena of the body that would be attributed to the "soul" and even the "nafs" and is something that permeates the entire body but departs when a person dies, whereas the blood and form of the body remains.

In Traditional Chinese Medicine, it is believed that health is maintained when the blood and "qi" flow smoothly throughout the body. When there is stagnation or stasis this leads to disease which can be systemic, affecting the whole body, or local, affecting a particular organ or part of the body. Hijamah is particularly effective at relieving this "stasis" and acts to restore proper flow especially of blood but also of qi in the body or local region

Stagnation or stasis is not the only pathology however that Hijamah treats within TCM. In TCM there is a disease differentiation system called the 8 patterns. In this system it is determined whether a disease is internal or external, hot or cold, excess or deficient and yin or yang. This matrix is then used to determine the core nature of an illness.

When this system produces a pattern that is excess and heat related then Hijamah is indicated. Excess heat patterns include Internal pathologies such as blood heat, blood toxins, liver heat, heat rising up in the body, stomach fire, large intestine fire, heart fire etc. and can be effectively addressed by حجامة or bloodletting. These patterns are characteristically defined by their being an "internal", "excess", "hot" pattern of disease.

"External" excess heat patterns correspond with febrile infectious diseases and can also be effectively addressed by bloodletting. These include traditional Chinese medicine patterns such as invasion of wind-heat, toxic heat, spring warm etc.

Normally Hijamah is not indicated when it is deficient heat pattern of any type of cold pattern except where there is significant stagnation. If it is used in these cases only a small amount of blood is removed so as not to worsen the "deficiency" or "cold" aspect of the disease.

In terms of the deeper principles of yin and yang, bleeding can also be used in cases of blood deficiency. For these cases a small amount of blood is removed which then has the effect of stimulating blood production.

Hijamah's effects within the traditional Chinese medicine paradigm:

1. Invigorates the flow of qi and blood and releases blockages
2. Disperses local areas qi and blood stasis, as in cases of areas of pain or visible stasis such as evidenced by the presence of spider and/or varicose veins.
3. Drain excess heat and fire from the exterior parts of the body and various internal organs.
4. Brings down yang or heat which is rising in the body (that may cause high blood pressure, migraine headaches and even lead to stroke).
5. Treats emergency conditions characterized by excess heat, epilepsy and/or mania.
6. Removes fire toxins from the body.
7. Stimulates blood production.

In summary, Hijamah has the following effects in terms of traditional medical paradigms:

Impurities:

1. Removes impurities from the blood
2. Diverts and expels toxins and harmful impurities from the vital organs

Balance of humors:

3. Removes excess blood

Heat and inflammation:

4. Draws inflammation away from the deeper organs
5. Drains excess heat and fire from the exterior parts of the body and indirectly from various internal organs.
6. Brings down yang or heat which is rising in the body (that may cause high blood pressure, migraine headaches and even lead to stroke).
7. Removes fire toxins from the body.

Circulation of blood and qi:

8. Invigorates the flow of qi and blood and releases blockages, improves blood circulation
9. Disperses local areas of qi and blood stasis, as in cases of areas of pain or visible stasis such as evidenced by the presence of spider and/or varicose veins.

Emergency conditions:

10. Treats emergency conditions characterised by excess heat, especially where there is a mental component to the symptoms such as mania, delirium, epilepsy etc.

Stimulatory effects:

11. Stimulates blood production.
12. Assists the body's own healing abilities

Other effects:

13. Treats Sihr (black magic) and Nazr(Evil eye)

While the above effects are attributed to Hijama's uses and understanding in traditional medical paradigms, there is mounting scientific evidence to support them. Hijamah's effects based on this research will be discussed in the next section and then linked back to the effects above for a greater depth to the understanding and application of Hijamah.

Modern Medical Understanding of Hijamah

The modern medical paradigm, (which is only approximately 100 years old, beginning with the discovery of the first antibiotic in 1908), is based on different principles to traditional medicine. Though it evolved from the 4-humor theory and most drugs were and still are developed based on herbalism, modern medicine has come to define disease as based primarily on a number of distinct internal pathologies viz.:

1. Infection by a foreign organism
2. Autoimmune disorders where the body's immune system is not functioning properly
3. Genetic disorders
4. Circulatory and perfusion abnormalities (high blood pressure, ischemia etc)

In addition modern medicine is highly concerned with controlling and repairing:

1. Inflammation
2. Uncontrolled and haphazard growth of cells (as in cancer)
3. Structural deformity and injury
4. Biochemical anomalies (eg. hormonal imbalance, cholesterol markers etc.)

To a lesser extent modern medicine is also concerned with:

1. Nutrition (and states of malnutrition and nutrient deficiency)

2. Lifestyle factors

While this is not exhaustive and there are many specialties within modern medicine, they do form the foundation of medical treatment and philosophy.

Prior to 1950, bloodletting was commonly used in modern medicine for a myriad of ailments related to the above pathologies, nowadays the most common accepted use for modern bloodletting is for a hereditary iron-overload condition known as haemochromatosis. As iron builds in the patient's blood, it can have a negative impact on various areas of the body, including the heart and the joints. This can eventually lead to disease and organ failure. Bloodletting, done as phlebotomy or more often in the form of "blood donation", is applied as the main treatment for haemochromatosis, with patients having their blood taken at least once annually for life.

Hijamah however has more applications in modern medicine and the research and scientific understanding supports this, as will be demonstrated in the following pages.

Before doing so it is important to understand the difference in blood composition between blood removed via Hijamah while observing its rules and that removed by other means or methods.

Composition of the blood removed in Hijamah

The University of Damascus has conducted extensive studies on the effects of Hijamah as well as the difference in blood composition when blood is removed according to the principles of Hijamah and also against it. The following discussion is based on their research and expanded upon by myself for the benefit of the reader who may not be familiar with the medical terms and the implications of the findings.

The study first examined the nature of the blood removed where Hijamah is done according to its principles, viz:

1.For males over 20 or females after they have passed menopause,
2.In the latter part of the lunar month
3.In the spring and summer seasons,
4.In the early morning
5.In a fasting condition
6.On the upper back between the shoulder blades

When this blood is examined from the sites of incision before application of suction (so as not to alter the cell structure), the blood is found to have the following qualities:

1. The red blood cells were predominantly abnormal, including:

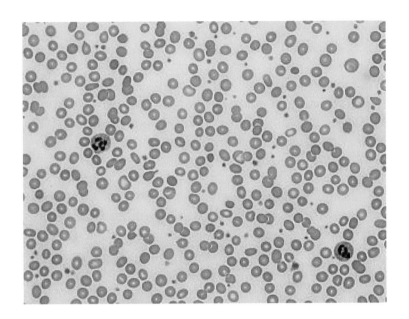

a. Hypochromic cells - these cells are normally seen in higher concentrations in patients with anemia, they appear paler than normal red blood cells. The concentration of these types of cells in healthy individuals is less than 5%. Blood removed in Hijamah however has a high number of these cells.

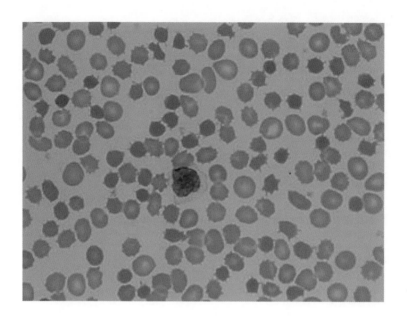

b. **Burr cells** - These cells are recognized by their irregular prickly shaped membrane (see above) and are regarded as aged red blood cells. Because these cells are regarded as "aged" red blood cells, they are not efficient in their function and there presence in the circulation diminishes the proper functioning of blood in the body. Hijamah blood tends to have more of these cells and when they are removed this leaves the remaining blood with a higher concentration of more efficient and younger red blood cells.

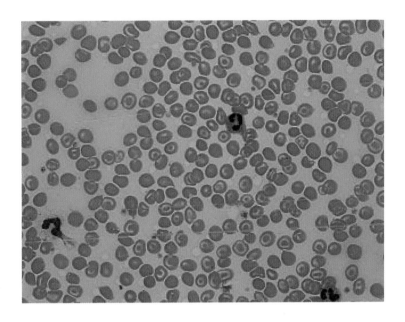

c. **Target cells** - (codocytes or leptocytes) have a "lump" of hemoglobinized cytoplasm within the area of normal central pallor, causing them to resemble a "bullseye" target. Target cells almost always indicate a pathological process when seen in higher than normal concentrations in regular blood samples. This is normally related to an imbalance between cholesterol and RBC ratios and may appear in association with the following conditions:

i. **Liver disease**

ii. Iron deficiency
iii. Thalassemias,
iv. Hemoglobin C diseases
v. Post-splenectomy: A major function of the spleen is the clearance of deformed, and damaged red blood cells. If splenic function

is abnormal or absent because of splenectomy, abnormal RBC's will not be removed from the circulation efficiently. Therefore, increased numbers of target cells may be observed.

2. The blood sample contained less white blood cells (525 to 950 per mm3) than found in general blood samples. In adult humans, the normal range of white blood cell counts is 4500 to 11 000 per mm3. This indicates that Hijamah while removing unhealthy and aged cells does not adversely affect the concentration of healthy white blood cells which are responsible for immune functions within the blood. Amongst the WBC, it was found that lymphocytes were of greater ratio, in the region of 52% to 88%. The significance of this is not yet clear.

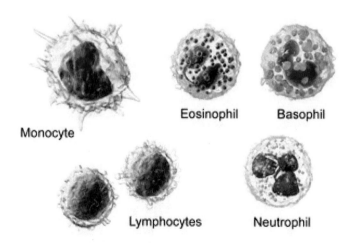

Monocyte

Eosinophil

Basophil

Lymphocytes

Neutrophil

White Blood Cells

3. TIBC is significantly raised in the blood sample and indicates a very high level of transferrin present in the Hijamah blood. This may be the reason why TIBC levels are normalized in the general blood after Hijamah is performed but requires further study to elucidate its full significance. Studies have showed that high transferrin saturation in the blood is correlated with increased incidence of cancer. Hijamah therefore may be playing an important role in cancer prevention as it acts to remove a larger proportion of transferring than is present in regular blood samples or blood donation.

4. Creatinine levels are high in the Hijamah sample. This substance is a breakdown product of creatine phosphate in muscle, and normally cleared from the body by the kidneys. Hijamah seems to assist in reducing the creatinine load and thereby help "detox" the blood of this substance.

5. The plasma ratio of the Hijamah blood was approximately 20%, indicating that the process does not remove blood plasma detrimentally.

When Hijamah is done against its principles as defined above, the blood removed is of different composition and appears similar to normal venous blood, this includes when it is done on different areas of the body and out of its regular times but also in these two states that warrant special mention:

Below the recommended age

The Damascus study showed that the blood removed from younger males in Hijamah was more consistent with regular venous blood with regard to the concentration of RBCs and WBCs, the shape of RBCs as well as the levels of uric acid, cholesterol and triglycerides. The recommended age for Hijamah is above 20, though it is recommended even later than this since there are relatively less blood problems while young. This of course will depend on the individual and their particular constitution and symptoms.

On a full stomach

The study had similar findings when patients had eaten a full breakfast before having the Hijamah done. This is against the principles of Hijamah which should be done on an empty stomach since after eating the circulation is diverted to the digestive organs and away from the peripheral areas. This changes the composition of the blood removed from the Hijamah area between the shoulder blades and now it resembles normal venous blood. From anecdotal evidence many practitioners report adverse effects such as weakness, gastrointestinal upset etc when Hijamah is done on a patient who has eaten recently.

Circulatory system effects

Modern physiological understanding maintains that blood loss of less than 750ml does not have any significant physiological effect on the body and is similar to the effect of donating blood. The blood removed in the Hijamah procedure however is not the same as that lost in cases of hemorrhage due to injury or blood donation which involves phlebotomy. Studies conducted at the Damascus University in Syria observing 330 patients who received Hijamah show that upon removal of blood via performing Hijamah within its principles, the following circulatory effects were observed:

In cases of hypotension and hypertension, blood pressure returned to normal parameters - this is easily explained by the slight loss in blood volume. In the case of the individuals with hypertension the loss is not sufficient to cause vasoconstriction and results in a lower blood pressure, but in the case of hypotension, the slight loss of blood is sufficient to induce vasoconstriction and therefore increases the pressure to normal levels. There may also be other mechanisms at work involving biochemical markers.

Studies confirm that Hijamah has beneficial effects on vascular compliance and degree of vascular filling and can also reduce high blood pressure in the acute setting.

(Note that the patient who is on blood pressure medication should not stop the medication after the Hijamah procedure, this may lead to a rebound effect

with dangerously high blood pressure readings. It is better that the patient works with their doctor in adjusting the dosage of the medication based on the blood pressure results.)

Normalised ECG readings - In patients with ECG anomalies, the individual segments showed return to a more normal ECG pattern.

In another study published in the Chinese Journal of Physiology[1], the effects of Hijamah on hemodynamic parameters, arrhythmias and infarct size (IS) after myocardial ischemic reperfusion injury in male rats was studied. (Rats were induced into having a heart attack in the laboratory setting, infarct size is the size of the damaged area of heart muscle. Arrthymias are the improper rhythm of the heart which are common with heart attacks.)

Results show that Hijamah:

● **Reduced the infarct size after injury**- this effect was most significant where hijamah was applied more than once

● **Significantly reduced Ischemic induced arrhythmias**

(This study however did not show any change in the baseline heart rate or mean arterial blood pressure.)

---

[1] Cardiac effects of cupping: myocardial infarction, arrhythmias, heart rate and mean arterial blood pressure in the rat heart.
Shekarforoush S, Foadoddini M.
Chin J Physiol. 2012 Aug 31;55(4):253-8. doi: 10.4077/CJP.2012.BAA042.

Effects on blood markers

ESR

The erythrocyte sedimentation rate (ESR) is the rate at which red blood cells sediment in a period of one hour. It is a common blood test, and may be an indicator of general inflammation. The ESR is increased by any cause or focus of inflammation and also in pregnancy, inflammation, anemia or rheumatoid arthritis and means that the red blood cells have a higher propensity of sticking together. It is also a diagnostic indicator for diseases such as multiple myeloma, temporal arteritis, polymyalgia rheumatica, various auto-immune diseases, systemic lupus erythematosus, rheumatoid arthritis, inflammatory bowel disease and chronic kidney diseases.

The Syrian Hijamah study showed that after Hijamah, ESR rates were lower in patients who previously had high ESR readings.

RBC count and Hb

In both cases of polycythemia where the red blood cell count is high and cases of low red blood cell count, there was a significant moderation of RBC count closer to normal values. It is already a well known treatment to use phlebotomy in patients with polycythemia but the effect of raising RBC count through bloodletting is unheard of. This can be explained by a stimulation of erythropoiesis, or red blood cell production in the body subsequent to Hijamah.

Hemoglobin levels also improved after Hijamah and may be related to the reduction of transferrin as mentioned

Thrombocytes

Thrombocyte levels were also moderated after the Hijamah procedure. In 50% of cases there was return to normal levels from either thrombocytosis or thrombocytopenia. This indicates that Hijamah has a beneficial effect for clotting problems.

Cholesterol and Triglycerides

In the Damascus study, subsequent to the Hijamah procedure, noticeable decreases in cholesterol and triglyceride levels were observed in more than 75% of patients who exhibited high levels before Hijamah. These indicators are associated with increased risk of heart disease and therefore suggest that Hijamah can reduce the risk of heart disease when done correctly.

The Iranian Society of Hijamah Research conducted further studies[2] into this effect, the aim of the study was to determine if a there was a reduction in serum lipoproteins via Hijamah, especially LDL cholesterol, and whether it is therefore a preventive approach against atherosclerosis.

In this trial, 47 men (18 to 25 years old), without chronic disease or a history of hyperlipidemia and

---

[2] J Altern Complement Med. 2007 Jan-Feb;13(1):79-82.

antihyperlipidemic drug consumption were randomly assigned into control and treated groups. Men in the treated group were subjected to Hijamah, whereas men in the control group remained untreated. The serum concentrations of lipids, collected from brachial veins, were determined at the time of Hijamah and then once a week for 3 weeks. The results showed a substantial decrease in LDL cholesterol in the treated group compared to the control. There were no significant changes in serum triglyceride between the groups however. The study concluded that Hijamah may be an effective method of reducing LDL cholesterol in men and consequently may have a preventive effect against atherosclerosis.

Glucose

Blood glucose levels were reduced in more than 80% of cases in the Damascus study. Of those who were diabetic, 92,5% experienced this reduction. Other studies also show improvement in metabolic syndrome.[3]

Metabolic syndrome is a term used to describe the list of medical problems facing people who are obese, such as hypertension, insulin resistance and glucose intolerance. People with this condition are at risk for clots and strokes. Bloodletting can help to prevent these problems though care should be taken

---

[3] The effects of wet cupping on coronary risk factors in patients with metabolic syndrome: a randomized controlled trial.
Farahmand SK, Gang LZ, Saghebi SA, Mohammadi M, Mohammadi S, Mohammadi G, Ferns GA, Zadeh MG, Razmgah GG, Ramazani Z, Ghayour-Mobarhan M, Azizi H.
Am J Chin Med. 2012;40(2):269-77.

in bloodletting those areas with already compromised blood flow, such as the feet in diabetic patients.

Uric acid

Uric acid is a product of the metabolic breakdown of purine nucleotides in the body and its increased circulation in the blood can lead to gout. High levels are also associated with diabetes and the formation of kidney stones. In many instances, people have elevated uric acid levels for hereditary reasons, but diet may also be a factor. High intake of dietary purines (found in many meats), high fructose corn syrup, and table sugar can cause increased levels of uric acid.[4] Serum uric acid can also be elevated due to reduced excretion by the kidneys.

The Damascus study showed improvement in uric acid levels with more than two thirds of patients undergoing Hijamah showing a decrease. This effect was more prevalent in those who had higher than normal uric acid levels to begin with. While this is a complex condition requiring other interventions including dietary and lifestyle changes as well, this shows that Hijamah can at least improve symptoms and is especially useful when done over the site of pain in the case of gout.

---

[4] Cirillo P, Sato W, Reungjui S, et al. (December 2006). "Uric acid, the metabolic syndrome, and renal disease". J. Am. Soc. Nephrol. 17 (12 Suppl 3): S165–8

Liver enzymes

Liver enzymes including ALT, AST and ALP are indicative of liver damage when found in larger than normal concentrations in the blood[5]. These enzymes are lower after the Hijamah procedure and suggest a possibility of improved liver function and health post the Hijamah procedure. Albumin levels also returned to normal in the Damascus study.

5 Lee, Mary (2009-03-10). *Basic Skills in Interpreting Laboratory Data*. ASHP. pp. 259–. ISBN 978-1-58528-180-0. Retrieved 5 August 2011.

Effect of Hijamah on the organs and systems

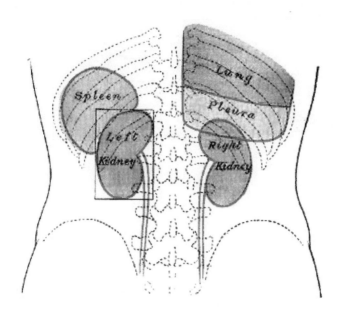

Hijamah has specific and general effects on the organs of the body and these are largely based on the indirect effects on circulation and altering of the blood composition described above. There are some direct effects however that relate to the area being bled and its connection with the particular organ

Spleen

The spleen is an organ in the body that acts as a blood filter—It removes old red blood cells and holds a reserve of blood in case of massive blood loss. It also recycles iron and has an important role in the function of the immune system. Disorders of the spleen include splenomegaly, where the spleen is enlarged for various reasons, such as cancer, specifically blood-based leukemias, and asplenia, where the spleen is not present or functions abnormally.

From the results of the composition of Hijamah blood, it is clear that Hijamah can reduce the load on the spleen by assisting in its function of removing aged blood cells and thereby assist with splenomegaly where it is due to congestion of the spleen due to inability to process large amounts of damaged or old RBCs. Hijamah is also necessary where the spleen has been removed.

Liver

The liver is a vital organ that has a wide range of functions in the human body, including detoxification, protein synthesis and production of biochemicals necessary for digestion. This organ plays a major role in metabolism and has a number of essential functions in the body, including glycogen storage, decomposition of red blood cells, plasma protein synthesis, hormone production, and detoxification. Because of its location and various functions, the liver is prone to many diseases such as

1. Infections such as hepatitis
2. Alcohol damage,
3. Fatty liver
4. Cirrhosis
5. Cancer
6. Drug damage

Many diseases of the liver are accompanied by jaundice caused by increased levels of bilirubin in the system. The bilirubin results from the breakup of the hemoglobin of dead red blood cells; normally, the liver removes bilirubin from the blood and excretes it through bile.

Because the liver can easily become overworked Hijamah has an effect on the liver similar to its effect on the spleen in that it reduces the work required by the liver in detoxifying the body and removing waste products. Hijamah therefore may assist in all the above liver diseases and also the resulting jaundice that may occur.

Kidneys

The effect on the kidneys is similar to that on the spleen. Hijamah assists the kidneys filtration function and lessens its load by removing impurities directly from the blood. After the procedure there is also heightened activity by the kidney in releasing erythropoietin which stimulates production of new red blood cells.

Nervous system

Anecdotal evidence shows that Hijamah is useful for both restoring proper blood flow to the brain (in cases of ischaemia) as well as reducing pressure in the brain when it is high. Hijamah may therefore be useful in the prevention and treatment of stroke, and it is also noted for its ability to improve memory and focus as reported by those who have had it done. (Treating stroke with Hijamah is an advanced method of Hijamah treatment and should not be done without proper training, it is discussed in detail in the Hijamah treatment guide for practitioners)

Effect of Hijamah on particular diseases

A number of studies have been conducted on the effect of Hijamah on particular illnesses and conditions. Exact treatment details on each disease are left for my practitioner level book but some research studies and reviews are described here for the benefit of the patient.

General research

1. The US Public Library of Science published a review in 2012 of all studies that examined the efficacy of cupping therapy. Only studies with randomized control trials were included in their analysis. What they were able to conclude after reviewing 135 experiments was that a) cupping therapy does not yield any serious adverse side effects, and b) cupping therapy was significantly better at improving patients' health when combined with other treatments compared to the other treatments alone. Combined therapy yielded more cured patients in these studies, especially those afflicted with shingles, facial paralysis (as with Bell's Palsy), acne, and spondylosis (or osteoarthritis of the neck)[6]

2. A systematic review published in *BMC Complementary and Alternative Medicine* in 2010 concluded that the majority of studies show

---

6 An updated review of the efficacy of cupping therapy.
Cao H, Li X, Liu J.
PLoS One. 2012;7(2):e31793. doi: 10.1371/journal.pone.0031793. Epub 2012 Feb 28.
Review.

potential benefit for pain conditions, herpes zoster and a number of other diseases.[7]

These studies confirm that Hijamah does not have adverse effects when done properly and more importantly confirms that it is indeed therapeutic in nature.

Diabetes

Recent studies conducted by Unani Practitioners in India[8] show that when Hijamah is combined with other therapies for Diabetes Mellitus, effectiveness of the therapy is increased in the treatment group. Hijamah was administered every month on the 17th day of the lunar calendar in keeping with the "Hijamah in Strength" principles. Symptoms such as polydipsia, polyphagia and polyuria were more improved in the treatment versus control group. The treatment group also showed improvement in wound healing, and lower blood glucose and cholesterol levels.

This study confirms the findings of the Damascus study showing that blood glucose (and cholesterol) levels are improved with Hijamah and therefore should be combined with regular therapies for the treatment of Diabetes Mellitus. This of course should

---

[7] Clinical research evidence of cupping therapy in China: a systematic literature review.
Cao H, Han M, Li X, Dong S, Shang Y, Wang Q, Xu S, Liu J.
BMC Complement Altern Med. 2010 Nov 16;10:70. doi: 10.1186/1472-6882-10-70. Review.

[8] Efficacy of unani regimen- hijama ma'a shurt (wet cupping therapy) with oral unani formulation in the management of ziabetus shakri (type-ii diabetes mellitus)"- A clinical study
Shaikh Nikhat , Rafath Mehmooda, Shakir Jameel , Sufiyan Ahamad Ghawte , Masroor A Qureshi

be done in keeping with the principles and having Hijamah every month should only be done if the climate is conducive to it. Excessive amounts of blood should not be removed if it is a monthly practice.

Pain

Hijamah is very effective for pain conditions and is probably the most common indication for Hijamah in the clinic setting. Anecdotal evidence suggests all types of pain disorders are well treated by Hijamah with the practitioner using different points on the body depending on the presenting signs and symptoms. There are a number of studies that support this:

In a Korean study[9] Hijamah was found to be superior than heat packs in improving **neck pain**, function and discomfort in cases of neck pain due to computer work.

---

[9] J Occup Health. 2012;54(6):416-26. Epub 2012 Sep 1.
Cupping for treating neck pain in video display terminal (VDT) users: a randomized controlled pilot trial.
Kim TH, Kang JW, Kim KH, Lee MH, Kim JE, Kim JH, Lee S, Shin MS, Jung SY, Kim AR, Park HJ, Hong KE.

A few studies[10],[11] also show that Hijamah is better than regular therapies in the treatment of **lower back pain.** In these studies Hijamah was associated with clinically significant improvement post treatment and at 3-month follow-up. The group who received Hijamah had significantly lower levels of pain intensity, pain-related disability and medication use than the control group.

Headaches are also well treated by Hijamah[12]. In one study, 70 patients with chronic tension or migraine headache were treated with Hijamah. Three primary outcome measures were considered at the baseline and 3 months following treatment: headache severity, days of headache per month, and use of medication. The results of the study showed that, compared to the baseline, headache severity decreased by 66% following Hijamah treatment. Treated patients also experienced the 12.6 fewer days of headache per month and had less reliance on pain medication. Hijamah therefore has clinically relevant benefits for patients with headache.

10 The effectiveness of wet-cupping for nonspecific low back pain in Iran: a randomized controlled trial.
Farhadi K, Schwebel DC, Saeb M, Choubsaz M, Mohammadi R, Ahmadi A.
Complement Ther Med. 2009 Jan;17(1):9-15. doi: 10.1016/j.ctim.2008.05.003. Epub 2008 Jun 24.

11 Trials. 2011 Jun 10;12:146. doi: 10.1186/1745-6215-12-146.
Evaluation of wet-cupping therapy for persistent non-specific low back pain: a randomised, waiting-list controlled, open-label, parallel-group pilot trial.
Kim JI, Kim TH, Lee MS, Kang JW, Kim KH, Choi JY, Kang KW, Kim AR, Shin MS, Jung SY, Choi SM.Source:Korea Institute of Oriental Medicine, Daejeon, Republic of Korea.

12 The efficacy of wet-cupping in the treatment of tension and migraine headache.
Ahmadi A, Schwebel DC, Rezaei M.
Am J Chin Med. 2008;36(1):37-44.

Shingles pain is another area where research has verified the effects of Hijamah. In a review[13] of 8 randomised controlled trials to evaluate the therapeutic effect of Hijamah for herpes zoster, the studies showed that Hijamah was better than medication for Herpes Zoster, in terms of the number of completely cured patients, the number of patients with improved symptoms, and the incidence rate of post-herpetic neuralgia (pain). The combination of Hijamah with medication was significantly better than medication alone.

Researchers also investigated the effect of Hijamah on **Carpal Tunnel Syndrome**[14], 52 patients with neurologically confirmed CTS were randomly assigned to either a treatment group which received Hijamah or a control group that had an application of a heat pack. Hijamah patients were treated with a single application of wet cupping, and control patients with a single local application of heat within the region overlying the trapezius muscle. Patients were followed up on day 7 after treatment. The primary outcome, severity of CTS symptoms (VAS), had greater reduction in the Hijamah group than in the control group, other aspects were also more improved in the Hijamah group, including neck pain, functional disability and physical quality of life. The

---

13 Wet cupping therapy for treatment of herpes zoster: a systematic review of randomized controlled trials.
Cao H, Zhu C, Liu J.
Altern Ther Health Med. 2010 Nov-Dec;16(6):48-54.

14 Effects of traditional cupping therapy in patients with carpal tunnel syndrome: a randomized controlled trial.
Michalsen A, Bock S, Lüdtke R, Rampp T, Baecker M, Bachmann J, Langhorst J, Musial F, Dobos GJ.
J Pain. 2009 Jun;10(6):601-8. doi: 10.1016/j.jpain.2008.12.013. Epub 2009 Apr 19.

treatment was safe and well tolerated. The researchers concluded that Hijamah may be effective in relieving the pain and other symptoms related to Carpal Tunnel Syndrome.

Other diseases

Though Hijamah enjoys such wide and frequent use, it remains more popular in countries that do not regularly publish research studies in english accessible journals, as a result research is still sparse on other conditions though anecdotal evidence and my own personal experience suggest that Hijamah is also effective, especially when combined with other therapies for the following illnesses:

•Gynecological disorders, including amenorrhea, infertility, endometriosis etc
•Dermatological (skin) disorders, including eczema, dermatitis, acne
•Neurological disorders including stroke, spinal cord injury, certain types of epilepsy etc
•Gastrointestinal disorders, especially those characterised by inflammation, including gastritis, nausea and vomiting, some infectious conditions etc

Warning: Biomedical training in addition to special training in Hijamah is required in order to treat many of these illnesses mentioned above. Knowing how to perform general Hijamah while not being versed in the clinical medicine aspects of these illnesses can result in severe adverse effects, so too can not understanding how to use the advanced Hijamah techniques used in illness even though one may be a qualified and experienced doctor. Practitioners are requested to refer to the Hijamah guide for Practitioners for detailed information.

Taiba theory[15]

A novel scientific theory explaining the medical effects of Hijamah was proposed by Salah Mohamed El Sayed from the Department of Medical Biochemistry of the Suhag university in Egypt. This theory, termed Taiba theory, described in the May 2013 edition of the journal *Alternative and Integrated Medicine* is currently the most accurate scientific explanation of Hijamah's curative properties.

Salah named this theory "Taibah" theory after the city of the Nabi (SAW), Madinah Munawwara in present day Saudi Arabia. Taibah is one of the names of this peaceful and blessed city and it means "clean", "pure" or "excellent". It also refers the ability of Madinah to purify its inhabitants and because it removes from it those that are impure and of ill-intention.

In summary, Taibah theory explains that *Hijamah is a minor surgical excretory procedure and its effect is similar to the mechanism of excretory function via glomerular filtration of the kidney, as well as abscess drainage, by which pathological (disease causing) substances are removed from the body*. This theory will be described in more detail below as presented by *Salah* in his paper.

---

[15] El Sayed SM, Mahmoud HS, Nabo MMH (2013) Medical and Scientific Bases of Wet Cupping Therapy (Al-hijamah): in Light of Modern Medicine and Nabiic Medicine. Altern Integ Med 2: 122. doi:10.4172/2327-5162.1000122

There are a few stages in the Hijamah procedure; first a cup is applied with suction before any piercing of the skin is performed. The cup is then removed after which the skin is pierced and the cup reapplied in order to draw blood from the resulting incisions.

1.When negative pressure is applied to the skin surface the first time a cup (or horn) is applied, the skin surface is lifted up into the cup due to its viscoelastic nature. The local pressure around the capillaries present inside this pocket lifted into the cup decreases and causes increased capillary filtration and thereby collection of filtered fluids which include causative pathogenic substances (CPS), old and damaged red blood cells, in addition to lymph and interstitial fluid in the interstitial space of this pocket. Chemical substances, inflammatory mediators and nociceptive substances released bathe the nerve endings present in the pocket resulting in analgesia, while any tissue adhesions are broken adding to the pain relieving effect of Hijamah.

2.When the cups are removed, a dramatic local increase in blood flow occurs, termed reactive hyperemia.

3.At the next stage incisions are made, before the cup is reapplied. The incisions allow removal of the CPS and collected fluids mentioned above and prevent their reabsorption into the venous system. It also causes release of endogenous opioids that add to the analgesic effect.

4. The second application of the cup and resultant negative pressure is transmitted through the incisions and creates a pressure gradient that causes excretion of the collected fluids that contains the CPS into the cup. Aged blood cellular fragments, and molecules and particles smaller than the capillary pore sizes selectively pass through the capillary pores under the negative pressure effect, while intact blood cells (larger than the size of pores and fenestrae of skin capillaries) do not. This explains the preponderance of unhealthy RBC's in Hijamah blood. The negative pressure suction and also release of nitric oxide, helps to dilate local blood capillaries. *Salah* explains *this improves microcirculation, increases capillary permeability, increases drainage of excess fluids, increases lymph clearance and flow, decreases absorption at the venous end of capillaries, increases fluid filtration at both arterial and venous capillary ends, and increases fluid excretion (filtered fluids and interstitial fluids) which acts to treat blood congestion, improve blood and lymphatic capillary circulation and resolve tissue swelling (due to removal of CPS, noxious substances, prostaglandins and inflammatory mediators).*

The positive effects of this include:

1. Improving oxygen supply,
2. Enhancing tissue perfusion and cellular metabolism
3. Preserving underlying tissue structure
4. Modulating angiogenesis
5. Relieving muscle spasm
6. Restoring balance of the neuro-endocrine system

7. Improving neurotransmission
8. Exerting pharmacological potentiation
9. Restoring physiological homeostasis.

Salah advises that Hijamah should be done whenever excess CPS or fluids are to be excreted. This can be determined either by applying Hijamah in strength for the person whose constitution allows it or by using the principles of Hijamah in illness by assessing the patient through differential diagnosis.

Guidelines for performing Hijamah

This guide is meant primarily for the patient who is interested in Hijamah for themselves and as a primer for the medical practitioner who wishes to know more about the mechanism and scientific basis of Hijamah, as well as its contraindications, precautions and indications.

For this reason and so as not to encourage those without the proper training, I do not describe the actual procedures of Hijamah in detail, this is left to the Hijamah treatment guide for practitioners. The guidelines below however are important to implement whether you are a prospective patient or a practitioner of Hijamah and should be observed in order to gain the benefits of this treatment without exposing oneself or one's patients to unnecessary harm through it.

Who should practice Hijamah

Hijamah is regarded as an invasive medical procedure and more importantly is such a procedure where the skin is pierced and there is subsequent handling of body fluids. Any such procedure in medicine presents with a large number of risks when compared to procedures where the skin is not pierced and there is no handling of body fluids.

In recent years there has been a proliferation of dangerous infections that are transmitted easily through blood and body fluids. These include HIV,

Hepatitis B, Hepatitis C and Viral Hemorrhagic Fever. Since it is difficult to determine what infectious pathogens any given blood contains, and some blood-borne diseases are lethal, standard medical practice regards all blood (and any body fluid) as potentially infectious.

There are many cases where Hijamah has resulted in infection with the HIV and Hepatitis viruses, at least one documented HIV infection has occurred in Saudi Arabia and two documented cases reported in Iranian studies. *(The majority of cases go undocumented as the patients may not be aware that they have been infected and/or practitioners neglect to report adverse effects for fear of prosecution)*

Other risks of Hijamah are also inherent in terms of dealing with the effects of excessive blood loss *(which may occur due to hereditary disease or medication the patient is taking)*, incorrect piercing of the skin and subsequent damage to nerves or blood vessels, all of which can potentially be fatal for the patient. Improper handling and disposal of body fluids and sharps is also a common occurrence by those practicing Hijamah without proper training and presents a serious risk of spread of infection to other members of the community.

For this reason it is the opinion of many Ulama that **the Hajjaam must be an individual who has had biomedical training**, either a medical doctor or a qualified and registered practitioner of complementary medicine, or at least an individual who has received specific training in Hijamah and has also received with it training in human anatomy, physiology, general pathology, clinical medicine, clinical diagnostics, differential diagnosis, pharmacological interactions and how to properly handle body fluids and prevent infections.

Most countries have a register of individuals who are qualified to practice medicine, whether conventional or complementary, and amongst these there are those who have learnt and practice Hijamah. In some countries like the UK there are specific registers for practitioners of Hijamah and such individuals have received training in the safe application of the procedure. These should be the individuals who are first sought for having Hijamah done and if one is interested in practicing Hijamah then one should endeavor to learn it properly with its necessary biomedical prerequisites in order to gain such formal qualification and registration.

Individuals who practice Hijamah without the necessary qualifications are opening themselves up to prosecution by the law in their country should anything go wrong whether it be their own carelessness or by chance. Medical malpractice litigation is becoming more and more common and an unregistered practitioner has no support in such a case from any health council or registration body.

In the US the regulations regarding Hijamah only allow the following licensed professionals to practice;

• Physicians
• Physicians Assistants (PA)
• Advanced Practitioner Registered Nurse (APRN)

• Licensed Acupincturist (LAc)
• Phlebotomists-Only allowed to draw blood in lab setting.
• Paramedics-Allowed to draw blood or do incisions in emergency situations only.

Of course there are some countries where the law is not strict about such matters, but the practitioner will have to live with the consequences of their lack of knowledge and experience in medical matters should something go wrong while practicing Hijamah.

Many believe that Hijamah is exclusively an Islaamic practice and therefore it should be legalised for any Muslim to practice it. This is erroneous since Hijamah is a medical practice that was already present before the coming of the Nabi (SAW) and was encouraged by the Nabi (SAW), it is not specific to any particular religion or culture but rather it is a treatment for the entire world. Unlike the use of honey and black seed, Hijamah is a **medical procedure** and because in Islaam we are taught to take precaution and not engage in anything that can cause harm to us both spiritually and physically, one should seek out an expert in Hijamah, who also has the necessary biomedical qualifications for the procedure.

(A list of individuals who have been assessed as having the necessary education and suitable qualifications can be found here: www.hujjaam.com, if you are a practitioner you can also go to the site to apply for assessment of your credentials and submission to the list)

General contraindications and precautions

As is discussed above, Hijamah is not without its risks, and it is not for everybody to undertake. The Hajjaam must see that the patient is fit for Hijamah and must know how to adapt the procedure based on the constitution of the patient and their current state of health. This is also borne out by the hadith:

*Jabir bin Abdullaah (RA) relates that he heard Rasulullaah (SAW) saying: "If there is any good in your treatments it is in the blade of the Hajjaam, a drink of honey or branding by fire (cauterisation/ moxibustion), **whichever suits the ailment**, and I do not like to be cauterized" (Bukhari & Muslim)*

This hadith infers that one must know if Hijamah is the best treatment for the patient, or another treatment would be more suitable. It is interesting to note that in this same hadith the 3 main principles of treatment are referred to, viz, supplementing (with honey), draining heat (by Hijamah) and treating cold and stasis (with fire).

In order to know if Hijamah will suit the patient the Hajjaam must first know the contraindications and precautions for practicing Hijamah. Contraindications being those conditions if present, in which Hijamah should not be done and precautions being those in which it is not prohibited, but caution should be observed, especially in terms of how much blood is removed.

Excessive perspiration

"Do not bleed the one who is sweating, do not sweat the one who is bleeding"

The first rule of preventing adverse effects of Hijamah is not to perform the procedure for a person who is suffering from excessive perspiration. In traditional medicine this is understood as a weakness of the body in its ability to hold the pores closed, which therefore results in excessive and easy perspiration. (This should not be confused with night sweats which are a different phenomenon mostly due to heat forcing the pores open at night.)

A person who suffers from easy and excessive sweating is already suffering from a loss of body fluids and bleeding such a person will only aggravate this condition. They will also tend to bleed more easily and may exhibit excessive and uncontrolled blood loss should Hijamah be performed. Excessive sweating, or hyperhidrosis, can be a warning sign of thyroid problems, diabetes or infection. It is also more common in people who are overweight or out of shape. Such an individual is not normally suffering from an "excess heat" type of condition where Hijamah is indicated.

The second part of this precaution, viz. do not sweat the one who is one bleeding, means that medication which is used to cause sweating (diaphoretics) should not be used in a person who is bleeding (as it will increase blood loss unnecessarily).

Hemophilia

Hemophilia is a genetic disorder that impairs the body's ability to control blood clotting or coagulation, which is used to stop bleeding when a blood vessel is broken, or to heal the incision that is created by the Hajjaam. It is more common in males than females and is characterized by lower blood plasma clotting factor levels of the coagulation factors needed for a normal clotting process. Thus when a blood vessel is injured, a temporary scab does form, but the missing coagulation factors prevent fibrin formation, which is necessary to maintain the blood clot. A hemophiliac does not bleed more intensely than a person without it, but can bleed for a much longer time. In severe hemophiliacs even a minor incision from Hijamah can result in blood loss lasting days or weeks, or even never healing completely. For this reason it is not recommended to perform Hijamah on a hemophiliac, unless it is in association with their medical practitioner who understands the severity and nature of the patients hemophilia and regards Hijamah as safe for the patient.

The Hajjaam should take a proper history of the patient in order to determine if the patient is a hemophiliac.

Anticoagulant drugs

If a patient is on medication, the Hajjaam must determine whether it is safe to continue with Hijamah and that the medication will not cause excessive and potentially uncontrollable bleeding or other adverse effects.

Amongst these medications the most dangerous are anticoagulant medicines. Anticoagulants are medicines that prevent the blood from clotting as quickly or as effectively as normal. Some people call anticoagulants blood thinners. However, the blood is not actually made any thinner - it just does not clot so easily whilst you take an anticoagulant.

Anticoagulants are commonly used to treat and prevent blood clots that may occur in your blood vessels. Blood clots can block an artery or a vein. A blocked artery stops blood and oxygen from getting to a part of your body (for example, to a part of the heart, brain or lungs). The tissue supplied by a blocked artery becomes damaged, or dies, and this results in serious problems such as a stroke or heart attack. A blood clot in a large vein, such as a deep vein thrombosis (a clot in the leg vein), can lead to serious problems such as a pulmonary embolism (a clot that travels from the leg vein to the lungs).

Patients on anticoagulant medication may exhibit excessive blood loss after Hijamah which in some cases can be fatal. The most common anticoagulants include warfarin and heparin, however these may go by different brand names and for this reason a Hajjaam should be familiar with basic pharmacology and be able to recognize anticoagulant use in prospective Hijamah patients. If you are using anticoagulants you should consult with your doctor before having Hijamah done.

If you are not sure whether you are using anticoagulant medication you can check your medication against this list of common names for anticoagulant medication, the list is not exhaustive and ideally your Hajjaam should have the knowledge and training to identify if you are using an anticoagulant or not:

Warfarin - Coumadin, Jantoven, Marevan, Lawarin, Waran, Warfant

Dabigatran - Pradaxa

Acenocoumarol - G 23350, Nicoumalone, Nicumalon

Phenindione - Dindevan, Fenindion, Phenylin-Zdorovye, Soluthrombine

Rivaroxaban - Xarelto

Note: Aspirin also has an effect of preventing clots by preventing platelets sticking together. However, it is classed as an antiplatelet agent rather than an anticoagulant.

Anemia

Anemia is a common condition in which the blood lacks adequate healthy red blood cells. Red blood cells carry oxygen to the body's tissues. Iron deficiency anemia is due to insufficient iron. Without enough iron, the body cannot produce enough hemoglobin, a substance in red blood cells that enables them to carry oxygen. As a result, iron deficiency anemia may leave an individual tired and short of breath.

A number of recent studies[16],[17] are showing a link between excessive and unnecessary bloodletting and iron deficiency anemia, some even as severe as resulting in cardiomyopathy which is only seen in chronic severe iron deficiency anaemia.[18]

For this reason care should be taken not to cause this type of anemia through Hijamah. This will most often occur when women who are menstruating normally receive Hijamah without a serious reason, or when Hijamah is practiced too often and/or too much blood is removed.

For the healthy person not living in a very hot climate, to have Hijamah once a year in the hot season is sufficient, provided the person exhibits signs of a healthy constitution and does not already suffer from anemia. If so, then it should be administered in a "low dose" only once every few years so as to encourage haematopoiesis. *(For a women who is menstruating general Hijamah is not needed except where the woman is suffering from an*

[16] Anaemia and skin pigmentation after excessive cupping therapy by an unqualified therapist in Korea: a case report.
Kim KH, Kim TH, Hwangbo M, Yang GY.
Acupunct Med. 2012 Sep;30(3):227-8. doi: 10.1136/acupmed-2012-010185. Epub 2012 Jun 27.

[17] A prospective evaluation of adult men with iron-deficiency anemia in Korea.
Yun GW, Yang YJ, Song IC, Park KU, Baek SW, Yun HJ, Kim S, Jo DY, Lee HJ.
Intern Med. 2011;50(13):1371-5. Epub 2011 Jul 1.

[18] Bloodletting-induced cardiomyopathy: reversible cardiac hypertrophy in severe chronic anaemiafrom long-term bloodletting with cupping.
Sohn IS, Jin ES, Cho JM, Kim CJ, Bae JH, Moon JY, Lee SH, Kim MJ.
Eur J Echocardiogr. 2008 Sep;9(5):585-6. Epub 2008 Jun 23.

abundance of blood as sometimes happens in the arab regions.)

Pregnancy

During pregnancy there is a tremendous demand by the baby for nourishment which is provided by means of the mothers blood. For this reason the woman's appetite grows tremendously due to the increased production of blood in her body. This is the system that Allaah has created to provide for the child in the womb of the mother. The heat of the body is also concentrated internally during the pregnancy period which leaves the outer parts relatively cold and lacking in blood. The normal menstrual cycle also ceases, which in traditional medicine is seen as a sign that there is no need for the woman to lose blood in this period. As a result, if Hijamah is applied in such a stage then great harm is done to the body and to the developing baby, this can easily result in miscarriage.

It is shocking to me when I hear that women who are pregnant are having Hijamah done, and on more than one occasion I have come to know that this has resulted in miscarriage. The irresponsible Hajjaam then hides behind the claim of "taqdeer" when in fact this is medical malpractice and they will be held responsible in the court of Allaah for not adhering to basic medical guidelines in respect of care during pregnancy.

Pregnancy is a clear contraindication for Hijamah, it should not be done or even considered during pregnancy and should a Hajjaam either due to ignorance or pursuit of money cause a miscarriage then the Hajjaam is to blame and in my opinion should be charged with a crime by the legal system prevailing in that country.

Wound healing disorders

When performing Hijamah incisions are made in the skin to release blood. Normally these heal within a short period and leave minimal scarring (especially when a post Hijamah blood and healing herbal formula and/or low level laser therapy is applied afterward).

In some conditions however, the body's ability to heal and repair the incision is impaired, and results in either a longer healing time, no healing at all or excessive scarring and keloid formation.

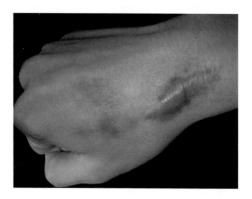

Example of Keloid formed after an operation due to a motorcycle accident

Keloids are thickened scars due to excessive synthesis of collagen after an acute injury, which can include the incision, required for Hijamah. Hypertrophic scarring and keloids most frequently arise in young adults and are particularly prevalent in dark-skinned individuals. They are equally common in males and females. These scars may also itch and/or be painful to touch. They are firm or hard, skin-coloured to bright red, smooth, elevated nodules and may have claw-like extensions far beyond the original wound. They are particularly frequently seen on earlobes, shoulders, upper back and anterior chest. Hijamah should be avoided in individuals who have a history of easily developing keloids and hypertrophic scarring. (This is not a contraindication but rather a precaution as we have experienced less occurrence of keloids if the patient is exposed to low level laser therapy after the procedure)

Healing of the incisions can also be impaired by other factors that slow down or prevent complete healing and include issues such as the lack of growth factors, the presence of edema, poor blood flow, infection, hypoxia, arterial or venous insufficiency and neuropathy.

Other systemic causes of impaired wound healing include metabolic disease, diabetes mellitus, the patients nutritional state, a history of smoking or drug use, exposure to radiation, aging, immune disorders, and abnormal collagen syndromes. A thorough history will reveal if the patient may have wound healing problems.

Diabetes deserves special mention as it is a common disorder and when present gives rise to a high risk of major complications in the Hijamah incision, including infection and cellulitis and can even lead to amputation when performed on the extremities. Vascular, neuropathic, immune function, and biochemical abnormalities in diabetes each contribute to delayed healing. Even careful wound care in a patient with excellent glucose control may fail and result in these adverse effects. Special care should therefore be taken in diabetic patients in order to determine whether Hijamah is appropriate for the patient and if so, it should be done only in those areas and in a way that will not risk poor wound healing, subsequent infection and other adverse effects.

Who should have Hijamah done

In the hadith related by Jabir ibn Abdullaah (RA), the Nabi (SAW), said: توافـق الـداء meaning "whichever fits the ailment", in these 2 words the entire field of differential diagnosis and differential treatment was proven and emphasised. In this particular hadith the Nabi of Allaah (SAW) said this in respect of the 3 treatments of honey, hijamah and cauterisation. This indicates that albeit established that the contraindications are not present and the precautions are observed, Hijamah may not be the appropriate treatment for the patient.

In order to determine if Hijamah fits the patient and their ailment the Hajjaam should possess some basic skills of differential diagnosis. This includes both western and traditional medicine diagnostic skills in order to determine two essential aspects, viz:

● The constitution or body type of the patient
● The pattern of the illness

Being able to determine these two aspects will guide the Hajjaam as to whether Hijamah fits the ailment or not.

Constitutions or body types

Hippocrates said that: "It is more important to know what sort of person has a disease, than to know what sort of a disease a person has."

This principle has all but completely departed from the practice of modern medicine but still remains an integral part of the practice of traditional medicine like Unani-Tibb and TCM. It is perhaps the most important criteria in both the identification of the nature of the disease as well as the selection of a treatment method. Understanding the type of person, their temperament as well as their lifestyle, social and environmental influences and history can make the difference between a successful resolution of the presenting illness and a litany of inaccurate diagnoses and ineffective treatments.

Recognising the body types is not difficult to master. There are 4 primary constitutions or body types within the Unani philosophy and 5 within the Traditional Chinese Medicine philosophy. These can be combined into 5 main body types for the purposes of determining the suitability of Hijamah. They are as follows:

Fire constitution (Hot and Moist - Sanguinous)

They have a strong circulatory system and manifest with red facial hues. These individuals have a hotter temperament, their build is large with more muscle, the skin is warmer, their complexion is reddish in colour and glowing, and the veins are prominent. They usually have broad paravertebral muscles and well-proportioned shoulders, upper back and thighs. Their head is smaller and somewhat pointed, with a pointed chin, small hands and feet and usually curly hair, often these individuals may have an early receding hairline.

They suffer from excessive thirst and are uncomfortable in the hot season. They tend to wear less clothing than others do and will sleep with the windows open. They may also be short in stature (dynamite in a small package) and have an "explosive" personality and tend to excessive laughter, they are persuasive, sociable, outgoing, talkative, all embracing, affectionate, expansive, generous, intuitive, warm and bright. Fire personalities are trusting, open minded, social, and fond of beauty. They are spontaneous and often funny.

Potential disorders they may suffer from include insomnia, arrhythmias, paranoia, restlessness, palpitations, nervous exhaustion, anxiety, agitation.

Wood constitution - (Hot and Dry - Bilious)

They have softer skin, more fat, medium to muscular body with prominent veins. They are resourceful, outspoken, and may be short-tempered.

Other words that describe them may include forceful, determined, bold, decisive, clear, tendency to overdo, over direct, over perform.

They also have small and shapely hands and feet, broad shoulders and a straight flat back. By nature these individuals enjoy the spring and summer seasons and tend to dislike autumn and winter, as their constitution leaves them more vulnerable to pathogenic invasion and disease during these seasons. They have strong sinews and tendons and tend to manifest with green bluish facial hues.

Wood constitutions tend to be kind, merciful, creative, and free in self-expression. They can also manifest stubbornness, dominance and may have issues with anger, excessive aggressiveness and are almost always overachievers. When sick they can be unassertive, unsure of themselves and their role in life. They may experience difficulties in expressing themselves, and have weak boundaries, and display timidity and self-doubt.

Potential disorders include blood glucose issues, PMS, muscle pains, allergies and hayfever, depressive episodes, epilepsy, intolerance, impatience, vascular o rmigraine headaches, They may also suffer from diarrhea and frequent indigestion.

Metal constitution (Cold and Dry - Melancholic)

Their skin is dry and rough, they are more slender than the average, appear thin and bony and dont put on weight easily even though they may have a voracious appetite, they do not tolerate dry foods. They like moist things, hot water and thin oils are readily absorbed by their skin. The complexion is sometimes described as greyish, sooty or otherwise they appear white and pale but not shiny, they tend to be thoughtful, logical, analytical, and are perfectionists. Other words that describe them include self restraint, methodical, efficient, and disciplined, lives according to principle, sense of symmetry, logical mind, purity of ideals.

Potential disorders include frequent Infections, chronic cough, COPD, sinus infections, dry skin, hair, skin disorders, stiff joints and muscles, shallow breathing, poor circulation.

Water constitution (Cold and Moist - Phlegmatic)

These individuals are often overweight and their skin feels cold to the touch. They have thin hair, a whitish shiny complexion, and laxity in the joints. In cold weather they become pale, leaden colored and have small veins. Their digestion is sluggish and often suffers from constipation. They tend to have a large round face, head and body, long upper back, large hips and may have uneven physical proportions.

They tend to be calm, accommodating, patient and good listeners.

Potential disorders include edema, urinary infections, impotence and infertility, low back weakness and pain, weak knees, deterioration of teeth, loss of libido.

Earth constitution

These individuals tend to have somewhat larger bodies and over proportioned head and abdomen, strong thighs, round face and wide jaw line. Their limbs are well proportioned and they often carry excess "flesh".

Balanced Earth personalities are predisposed to quiet peaceful lives unconcerned with wealth and fame. They are always at peace, calm and generous, forgiving and sincere. In life they are analytical, practical and logical with strong adaptability to changing circumstances.

Earth constitutions can develop digestive and gastrointestinal tract illnesses as these organs can get injured with excessive worrying and over thinking.

Qualities that describe an earth constitution include being practical, down-to-earth, intelligent, anticipating, meeting needs of the family, kind, supportive, pliant, reliable. They can sometimes however become too pushy and possessive.

Potential disorders include weight difficulties, obsessions, worry, self-doubt, digestive disturbances, low energy, cold limbs, food allergies, weak muscles, and unrealistic expectations, meddling, overprotective.

Constitutions suited to Hijamah

Of these only the Fire, Wood and to a lesser extent Earth constitutions are suited to regular Hijamah. These constitutions display an excess of either (liver/ heart) heat and blood in the case of the fire type, (liver) heat and stagnation in the case of the wood type, or stagnation and (stomach) heat in the case of the Earth type. They therefore benefit tremendously from Hijamah done as a general health preservation modality.

For the other constitutions, Hijamah is not generally indicated and if done must be done keeping in mind the principles of Hijamah done in illness. Too much blood must also not be removed as these individuals are already either deficient in blood (metal type) or deficient in heat (water type). There are times however when Hijamah applied in specific areas and for specific illnesses can be beneficial. This is described in further detail below:

8 patterns of illness

In TCM, one method of understanding the basic nature of an illness is to assess the ailment in terms of the "8 patterns". These are in fact 4 sets of opposing concepts viz.:

Hot / Cold
Internal / External
Excess / Deficiency
Yin / Yang

When determining if an illness is suited to treatment by Hijamah we are mostly concerned with 2 of these sets, viz. hot/cold and excess/deficiency. There are a number of ways to determine and differentiate how the ailment relates to these concepts such as through asking about the presenting symptoms, as well as looking at the tongue and feeling the pulse.

Pulse and tongue diagnosis are specialist fields that require practical training and therefore full detail is not provided on these aspects of diagnosis. Briefly, for Hijamah to be suitable for the ailment, the pulse should be rapid, floating or surging, not slow, deep or weak. it also should not be floating and hollow in the center. (For practitioners who want to explore the fascinating field of pulse diagnosis in detail I suggest signing up for my next course on pulse diagnosis here: www.pulsediagnosiscourse.com)

Asking about the symptoms in order to determine the nature of the illness is a method that is accessible to most and can provide enough information in the majority of cases to come to a diagnosis vis. a vie the pattern of illness.

When determining heat we differentiate between excess heat or deficient heat.

Excess heat has the following characteristics:

Main Signs: Fever (sometimes), thirst, red face, red eyes, constipation. Urine is scanty and dark.

Pulse: Rapid and Full
Tongue: Red with a yellow coating

The following are some general signs of an Excess Heat pattern though the exact symptoms depend on the organ(s) affected.

- Raised, red skin eruption that feels hot e.g. acute urticaria
- Any burning painful sensation e.g. urine or stomach pain
- Loss of blood with large quantities of bright red blood indicates Heat in the Blood
- Extreme mental restlessness/manic behavior (Heat in the Heart)
- Thick, yellow, sticky, malodorous secretions/ excretions

Excess Heat patterns are caused by excess of energy and blood in the body and individuals presenting with this type of pattern will respond very well to Hijamah.

Deficient heat has the following characteristics:

Main Signs: Afternoon fever or feeling of heat in afternoon, dry mouth, dry throat at night, night sweats, fever in 5 hearts, dry stools, scanty-dark urine, mental restlessness and fidgeting, vague anxiety. (More specific signs depend on Organ involved)

Pulse: Floating-Empty and Rapid or Thin and Rapid
Tongue: Red, in severe cases peeled. No Coating.

Other signs that may be present:

Deficiency heat affecting the Lung - Malar flush, dry cough.
Deficiency heat affecting the Liver - Headaches, dry eyes, irritability.
Deficiency heat affecting the Heart - palpitations, insomnia and feelings of restlessness.
Deficiency heat can be caused by many factors, stress being a major one. Excessive sexual indulgence, overwork, smoking, alcohol and drug abuse, all deplete the fluids and give rise to this type of heat as well. Long-standing emotional distress can also cause this pattern.

Such patients are suited to Hijamah but only with small quantities of blood removed. If the patient is suffering from excessive sweating then Hijamah is contraindicated.

Circulation issues

Irrespective of the constitution, circulation problems are well treated by Hijamah provided that the area affected is treated directly. In order to determine if the circulation is affected in a particular area of the body, the practitioner will have to take a thorough history and examine the area. Though full detail is beyond the scope of this book and must be learned through a course in clinical diagnostic skills in addition to other subjects, there are some signs that indicate poor circulation, viz:

● The are feels cold to the touch when compared to other areas
● There are prominent spider veins which appear purplish in nature.
● The patient experiences pain of a sharp and stabbing nature in the area
● There are purple spots on the tongue corresponding with the affected body area.

In these cases Hijamah may be beneficial though some special techniques must be employed such as bleeding of the spider veins etc. (This is detailed in the Hijamah Treatment Guide for Practitioners)

Geographical considerations

Modern medicine has not fully understood the effect of the climate on the health of individuals, yet traditional and complementary medical systems place tremendous emphasis on the climate, season and prevailing weather in the geographical area that a person resides in. Hakims are famous for recommending some patients move to another town or city that had a more favorable climate as the only method of treatment for the patients ailment. Similarly, the climate and weather must be taken into account when determining the suitability of Hijamah as is also borne out by this hadith:

*Anas ibn Maalik (RA) reported that the Rasul (SAW) said, "**When the weather becomes extremely hot, seek aid in Hijamah.** Do not allow your blood to rage (boil) such that it kills you." [Reported by Hakim in his 'Mustadrak' and he authenticated it and Imam ad-Dhahabi agreed (4/212)].*

From this we learn that Hijamah is suited to the hot climate, and this is corroborated by other Ahadeeth as well. If the patient lives in a region where the climate is normally hot, then Hijamah is probably suited to the patient. If the patient lives in a region where it is always cold, then care should be taken even if the patient displays the correct constitution for Hijamah. Every patient's condition will be different and it is up to the skilled and experienced Hajjaam to determine the weight of the climate, season and prevailing weather on the suitability of Hijamah. One may find that the season is correct, the dates are correct, the patient is suited to Hijamah but the particular weather on that day is cold and rainy. I would normally avoid doing Hijamah on such a day and postpone it to another day if it were a general Hijamah.

In the commentary on the books of Ahadeeth, Ulama have also written the following which must be considered:

"The saying of Sayyidina Rasulullaah SallAllaahu 'Alayhi Wasallam that cupping is the best medicine is very true. By this he was addressing the youth of the Haramayn, and also the inhabitants of the countries where the climate is hot, because their blood becomes thin, it remains more on the surface of the body and the climate of the country brings it even more closer to the surface."

The condition of the person having Hijamah

If Hijamah has been deemed suitable the patient must ensure to prepare themselves and be in the appropriate condition for the procedure. This is evident from a number of Ahadeeth such as the following:

*Ibn Umar (RA) reported that the Rasul (SAW) said, "**Hijamah on an empty stomach is best**. In it is a cure and a blessing..." [Saheeh Sunan ibn Maajah (3487)].*

Ibn Umar (RA) reported that the Rasul (SAW) said, "Hijamah on an empty stomach* is best. In it is a cure and a blessing. **It improves the intellect and the memory...**" [Saheeh Sunan ibn Maajah (3487)].

This is the most important condition, i.e. the **patient should have an empty stomach**.

The reason for this, especially in the case of Hijamah in strength, is because during the night, the toxins and impurities in the blood accumulate in the regions where Hijamah is done and remain there until a person eats. When a meal is taken blood is redirected to the digestive organs to enable the process of digestion and absorption. The toxins and impurities are therefore recirculated throughout the body instead of being concentrated in the Hijamah areas and also there is less blood in the superficial or outer parts of the body. If Hijamah is done in this condition it can lead to illness and this is also mentioned in some other Ahadeeth which say that Hijamah on a full stomach is disease and on an empty stomach is cure.

When Hijamah is done on a person who has just eaten it often results in vertigo or syncope (fainting).

The second condition is that the **person should have enough strength for the procedure**. This is also proven for the hadith:

The Nabi, upon whom be peace, was cupped while he was fasting. However, if doing this weakens the fasting person, it is disliked. Thabit al-Bunani asked Anas: "Did you dislike cupping for a fasting person during the time of the Nabi?" He answered: "No [we did not], unless it made someone weak." This is related by al-Bukhari and others.

There are some general conditions which are also recommended:

- The patient should ideally have taken a bath before the procedure, this assists in bringing the blood to the surface and helps it to flow better during the procedure.
- The are where Hijamah is to be done should be shaved, (often this will be done by the Hajjaam)
- The patient should give some sadaqah (charity) beforehand. It is recommended in the Ahadeeth to treat the sick with charity, it prevents calamities and in the case of the Hijamah procedure helps with the procedure being easy and successful.

When should Hijamah be performed?

Hijamah can be performed either in general cases (Hijamah in strength) when the patient is healthy or to treat a particular illness (Hijamah in illness). The times stipulated for these are different.

Hijamah in strength

For general health in those who are suited to cupping, it should be done once a year. During the Spring or Summer time when it is hot is the best season in which to perform Hijamah. The reasons have been described in previous chapters.

Hijamah and the lunar cycle:

In health it is generally recommended to perform Hijamah only on the 17th, 19th or 21st of the lunar month. These are the dates recommended in the Ahadeeth but there is no harm in doing it any time in the latter part of the lunar month from the 17th to the 27th, provided that the climate is suitable for it as detailed above.

The reason for this has to do with the effect of the moon on the blood. Just as the moon has an effect on the sea and produces high tides, in the same manner when the moon is full it brings forth impurities from the blood to the surface of the body and has other effects as well.

it is interesting to note that the term "lunatic" is derived from lunar and indicates the effect of the moon and such behaviour. In fact, lunacy is more likely at the time of the full moon since this is when there is a lot of liver energy which can give rise to easy anger, flared tempers etc.

Many who suffer from conditions such as epilepsy, migraine headaches, high blood pressure etc note that their symptoms are worse during a full moon that at other times of the month. Studies show that more assaults occur around the full moon. More crimes, self and unintentional poisonings and animal bites occur during the full moon cycle as well. The moon also has an impact on fertility, menstruation, and birth rate. Melatonin levels which are influenced by the phase of the moon correlate with the menstrual cycle. Admittance to hospitals and emergency units because of various causes also correlate with the moon phases. In addition, other events associated with human behavior, such as traffic accidents, crimes, and suicides, are more common during the full moon phase as well.

Studies indicate that melatonin and endogenous steroid levels are affected by the phase of the moon and may be the means by which the physiological changes occur in response to the moon phase. The release of these neurohormones may be triggered by the electromagnetic radiation and/or the gravitational pull of the moon.[19]

In a more recent study conducted in 2013 at the Psychiatric Hospital of the University of Basel,

---

[19] The lunar cycle: effects on human and animal behavior and physiology.
Zimecki M.
Postepy Hig Med Dosw (Online). 2006;60:1-7. Review.

Switzerland, researchers found that around the time of full moon, sleep was affected with subjects experiencing decreased electroencephalogram (EEG) activity, taking longer to fall off to sleep, and also reporting decreased sleep quality. This also correlated with lower melatonin levels.[20]

It is however not recommended to have Hijamah during the full moon phase itself, as it is understood that the blood will flow in excessive and unnecessary amounts, but afterwards (from the 17th onward) it is a means of removing the impurities and 'heat' from the body.

Time of day:

It is recommended to perform general Hijamah in the **early morning before 10 a.m.** while the impurities in the blood are still settled in the areas bled for Hijamah and have not had time to circulate and diffuse in the general circulation. Once the patient starts to get involved in his/her daily activities there is a significant redistribution of blood which is allocated to areas of the body that are in greater need depending on the activity being performed. The patient also may eat something which will cause blood to move to the internal digestive organs.

By the afternoon, the blood starts to recede internally and this is why "blood deficiency" headaches tend to occur at this time. Office workers are especially prone to this and should not be treated with Hijamah

---

[20] Evidence that the lunar cycle influences human sleep.
Cajochen C, Altanay-Ekici S, Münch M, Frey S, Knoblauch V, Wirz-Justice A.
Curr Biol. 2013 Aug 5;23(15):1485-8. doi: 10.1016/j.cub.2013.06.029. Epub 2013 Jul 25.

after returning from work as this aggravates their blood deficiency issue.

If the patient has had an afternoon nap and is fresh in the evening then Hijamah may be performed provided the climate is hot and the patient has not eaten.

Hijamah in illness

Hijamah in illness can be performed at any time of the month, but it is preferred during the daytime and when the climate is warm or hot. If this is not possible care should be taken that the room where Hijamah is being performed is warm and there is no draught entering, (whether it be through an incompletely sealed door or window etc.).

The patient should also take extra precaution not to expose themselves to cold after the procedure and neither should they drink or eat cold or raw foods as these will divert heat to the interior of the body. For Hijamah during illness the amount of blood removed must correspond with the level of the pulse and the Hajjaam must have special training in order to apply the procedure effectively to treat the presenting illness. It is better that the treatment is also combined with herbal medication and dietary therapy in such cases.

Body areas for Hijamah

For Hijamah in strength there are 3 main areas as mentioned above for the procedure. These are the head, the area between the shoulder blades and the on the anterior aspect of the foot.

Each of these is relevant to a different constitution though this is a guideline and not a rule.

The head area is more suited to the fire type constitution, the area between the shoulder blades to the wood type and the anterior aspect of the foot to the earth type who suffers from heat in the stomach.

These areas are also proven from the Ahadeeth:

*Anas bin Maalik RadiyAllaahu 'Anhu said: "Rasulullaah SallAllaahu 'Alayhi Wasallam used the treatment of Hijamah on both **sides of his mubaarak neck and between both shoulders, and generally took this treatment** on the seventeenth, nineteenth or the twenty first of the (lunar) month". (Tirmidhi 49:005)*

For Hijamah during illness, the points are not specific and will depend on the condition. The Nabi (SAW) also had this type of Hijamah done as borne out by the following Hadith:

*Anas bin Maalik RadiyAllaahu 'Anhu reports: "Sayyidina Rasulullaah SallAllaahu 'Alayhi Wasallam **took treatment of Hijamah on the back of his leg** at Milal (a place about seventeen miles-27 km-from Madinah Munawwarah in the direction of Makkah)* *while he was in the state of Ihraam". (Tirmidhi 49:006)*

(Further detail on the points used and the methods for Hijamah during illness is described in the Hijamah treatment guide)

Areas/points that should not be bled

There are a number of areas that should not be bled for the purpose of Hijamah. Some of these lie in close proximity to arteries; others are empirically not suited to bleeding therapies. These include the following areas:

Over the radial artery at the wrist

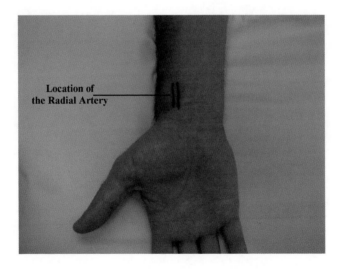

Over the axillary artery (in the armpit)

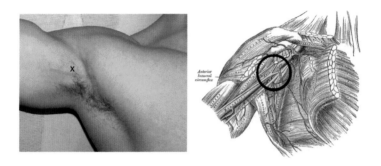

Over the posterior tibial artery

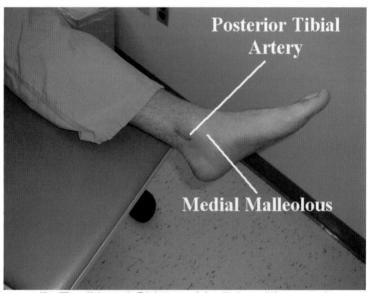

(In Traditional Chinese Medicine this area is connected to the kidney and bleeding here can be detrimental to kidney health)

Over the external iliac artery on the lower abdomen

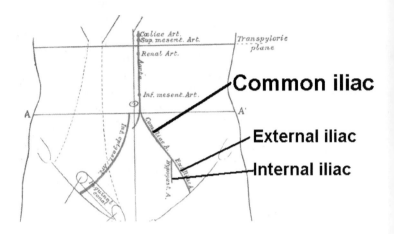

Over the carotid artery in the neck

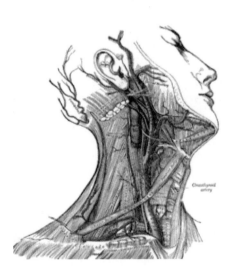

Some areas that overly arteries can be bled but caution must be taken when bleeding so as not to puncture the artery and cause excessive bleeding, these include the *dorsalis pedis* on the upper aspect of the foot, the *superficial temporal artery* located at the temples on the head.

How much blood should be removed?

In general Hijamah between 2 to 6 "cups" of blood are removed and this will depend on the constitution of the patient, their current state of health and the change in the color of the blood during the Hijamah procedure.

The constitution is determined as described earlier, with the fire type having the most amount of blood, followed by the liver and earth types.

Feeling the pulse is the best way to determine the current state of health. In general there are three levels of strength to the pulse, these can be described as forceless, normal force and forceful.

In terms of the color of blood, the range is from dark purplish to bright red.

Using these parameters one can determine the amount of blood to be removed in each case by following the table on the next page:

Constitution	Pulse strength	Cups
Earth	Normal	2
Earth	Forceless	0
Earth	Forceful	4
Wood	Normal	4
Wood	Forceless	2
Wood	Forceful	6
Fire	Normal	6
Fire	Forceless	4
Fire	Forceful	8

The third parameter is not used in the table as it overrides the other parameters, which means that If during the Hijamah procedure the blood changes from purple or dark red to a fresh or bright red, the procedure should be stopped and no further blood removed.

What to do after Hijamah?

There are a number of precautions that must be adhered to after the Hijamah procedure. These are essential to prevent infection and also to avoid adverse effects that may occur after the treatment.

The incisions should be cleaned and disinfected appropriately and thereafter covered with a suitable dressing or plaster. I also recommend the use of low-level laser therapy over the incisions to reduce the likelihood of scarring and speed up healing.

The body is in a condition of vulnerability after Hijamah and care must be taken to avoid exposure to cold as well as the weakness that arises from not eating appropriately after Hijamah. For this reason it is recommended to cover the body appropriately after Hijamah especially if the weather may be cold or damp. There is also the possibility of blood clots developing if the patient remains immobile afterward, one should therefore not go to sleep immediately afterwards but rather take a short walk and remain active for a few hours before resting.

Recommended foods include those that are rich in healthy fats and proteins and these should be taken one hour after the Hijamah. Plenty of fluids should be taken to redress the loss of body fluids, but refrain from caffeine and sugary drinks. I recommend a herbal formula which I personally developed called *HHT*, it is specifically formulated for use after Hijamah. The formula is a blood tonic that encourages production of new healthy blood, prevents adverse effects that may occur after the treatment including headaches, weakness, fatigue etc. and also strengthens the vital organs such as the kidneys, spleen and heart. It is available from www.aconitemedical.com/collections/hijamah

Hijamah patients should also avoid showering immediately after the procedure and take care not to scratch the incisions as this will contribute to scarring. The dressing should be changed daily or as needed until the wound has completely healed.

The practitioner should dispose of the instruments used and the blood in an appropriate manner to avoid cross infection. Many cases of Hepatitis and HIV have been reported as a result of mishandling of medical waste. The ideal situation is that the cups used are buried irrespective of whether they are glass or plastic cups. It is possible to sterilise glass cups but the preference would still be to bury them or dispose of them in special medical waste disposal facilities. Prospective patients can also take their own cups to the Hajjaam to ensure that Hijamah is not being administered to them using cups that were used on other patients before them, these are also available at www.aconitemedical.com/collections/hijamah.

Conclusion

In concluding this book I want to repeat that Hijamah is a healing method proven from the Ahadeeth and validated by medical science and scientific research. It should be sought out by those suffering from both common as well as rare illnesses, provided that the Hajjaam is qualified to assess and conduct the treatment correctly.

A listing of qualified and responsible Hujjaam is available at www.hujjaam.com.

Prospective Hijamah patients should take responsibility for their own healthcare and ensure they understand their own constitution and a bit about their illness before choosing Hijamah. If it seems indicated then there can be no better treatment. But if Hijamah is not suited to the ailment, it is unwise to insist on having Hijamah done or to see a Hajjaam who does not discriminate on who is given the treatment.

The author humbly requests your sincere duaas, may Allaah make this endeavor a means of khair and benefit for the ummah and may He grant me the ability to continue writing works that are of benefit.

Jazakamullaah
Dr Feroz Osman-Latib

Follow me for updates: www.DrLatib.com Twitter: @DrLatib or find me on Facebook: DrLatib

A note on copyright in Islam

It has become a common practice nowadays amongst Muslim readers to ignore copyright under the false assumption that such a concept does not exist in Islam. This has affected many authors ability and inclination to continue producing good works that benefit the Ummah and for this reason I am compelled to reproduce Mufti Taqi Usmani's writing on the subject:

"The question of "copyright" is related to a wider concept, generally known as the concept of "intellectual property". In previous days the concept of ownership was confined to those tangible commodities only which can be perceived through our five senses. But the speedy progress in the means of communication gave birth to the new concept of "intellectual property" which extended the concept of ownership to some intangible objects also.

The theory of "intellectual property" contemplates that whoever applies his mental labour to invent something is the owner of the fruits of his labour. If a person has invented a certain instrument, he does not own that instrument only, but he also owns the formula he has used for the first time to invent it. Therefore, nobody can use that formula without his permission. Similarly, if a person has written a book, he is the exclusive owner of the right to publish it, and nobody has any right to publish that book without his permission. This right of an author or an inventor is termed as his "intellectual property". It is also implied in this theory that the owner of such rights can sell them to others like any other tangible objects. The law of "copyright" has come into existence in order to secure such rights and to give legal protection to this kind of property.

It is obvious that the concept of intellectual property on which the law of copyright is based is a new phenomenon created by the rapid progress of industry and the means of communication; therefore, the concept is not expressly mentioned in the Noble Qur'an or in the Sunnah of the Blessed Nabi (S.A.W).

The acceptability or otherwise of such new concept which are not clearly mentioned in the original resources of Islamic jurisprudence can only be inferred from the general principles laid down by the Shari'ah. As the views of the jurists may differ while applying these principles to the new situations, there is always a wide scope of difference of opinion in such cases. The question of "intellectual property" has also been a subject of discussion among the contemporary Muslim scholars of Shari'ah whose opinions are different about its acceptability in Shari'ah.

A group of contemporary scholars do not approve the concept of "intellectual property". According to them the concept of ownership in Shari'ah is confined to the tangible objects only. They contend that there is no precedent in the Noble Qur'an, in Sunnah or in the juristic views of the Muslim jurists where an intangible object has been subject of private ownership or to sale and purchase. They further argue that "knowledge" in Islam is not the property of an individual, nor can he prevent others from acquiring knowledge, whereas the concept of "intellectual property" leads to monopoly of some individuals over knowledge, which can never be accepted by Islam.

On the other hand, some contemporary scholars take the concept of "intellectual property" as acceptable in Shar'iah. They say that there is no express provision in the Noble Qur'an or in the Sunnah which restricts ownership to tangible objects only. There are several intangible rights accepted and maintained by the Shariah, and there are several instances where such intangible rights have been transferred to others for some monetary consideration.

They contend that the concept of "intellectual property" does in no way restrict the scope of knowledge, because the law of "copyright" does not prevent a person from reading a book or from availing of a new invention for his individual benefit. On the contrary, the law of "copyright" prevents a person from the wide commercial use of an object on the ground that the person who has invented it by his mental labour is more entitled to its commercial benefits, and any other person should not be allowed to reap the monetary fruits of the former's labour without his permission.

The author of a book who has worked day and night to write a book is obviously the best person who deserves its publication for commercial purposes. If every other person is allowed to publish the book without the author's permission, it will certainly *violate the rights of the author, and the law of copyright protects him from such violation of rights.*

Both of these views have their own arguments. I have analysed the arguments of both sides in my Arabic treatise "Discussion of Contemporary Legal Issues" and have preferred the second view over the first, meaning thereby that a book can be registered under the Copyright Act, and the right of its publication can also be transferred to some other person for a monetary consideration.

I would like to add that if the law of copyright in a country prevents its citizens from publishing a book without the permission of the copyright holder, all the citizens must abide by this legal restriction. The reasons are manifold.

Firstly, it violates the right of the copyright holder which is affirmed by the Shariah principles, according to the preferable view, as mentioned earlier.

Secondly, I have mentioned that the views of the contemporary scholars are different on the concept of "intellectual property" and none of them is in clear contravention of the injunctions of Islam as laid down in the Noble Qur'an and Sunnah. In such situations, an Islamic state can prefer one view over the other, and if it does so by specific legislation, its decision is binding even on those scholars who have an opposite view. It is an accepted position in the Islamic jurisprudence that the legislation of an Islamic state resolves the juristic dispute in a matter not expressly mentioned in the Noble Qur'an or in the Sunnah. Therefore, if an Islamic state promulgates a law in favour of the concept of "intellectual property" without violating any provision of the Noble Qur'an and Sunnah, the same will be binding on all its citizens. Those who have an opposite view can express their standpoint in academic discussion, but they cannot violate the law in practice.

Thirdly, even if the government is not a pure Islamic government, every citizen enters into an express or a tacit agreement with it to the effect that he will abide by its laws in so far as they do not compel him to do anything which is not permissible in Shariah. Therefore, if the law requires a citizen to refrain from an act which was otherwise permissible (not mandatory) in Shariah, he must refrain from it.

Even those scholars who do not accept the concept of "intellectual property" do not hold that it is a mandatory requirement of Shari'ah to violate the rights recognized by this concept. Their view is that it is permissible for a person to publish a book without it's author's permission. Therefore, if the law prevents them from this "permissible" act, they should refrain from it as their agreement (of citizenship) requires them to do so.

Therefore, it is necessary for every citizen to abide by the law of copyright unless it compels a person to do an impermissible act, or to prohibit him from performing a mandatory act under the Shari'ah."

The reality is that many authors rely on the income from the sale of their books to continue the time consuming work of researching and writing without the need to resort to other means of earning. Infringing on copyright by choosing to copy these books and distribute them without permission hinders the author's ability to produce further works and is no act of piety, rather it is another of the traps of Shaytaan who is deft at guising evil as good.

If this book has come to you by way of copyright infringement I urge you to buy a genuine copy, it is the right thing to do.

May Allaah give us all the taufeeq and understanding to follow the guidance when it comes to us. Aameen